MW00647671

Sexual Harassment

Recent Titles in
Q&A Health Guides

SEXUAL HARASSMENT

Your Questions Answered

Justine J. Reel

Q&A Health Guides

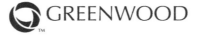

An Imprint of ABC-CLIO, LLC

Santa Barbara, California • Denver, Colorado

Library of Congress Cataloging-in-Publication Data

Names: Reel, Justine J., author.
Title: Sexual harassment : your questions answered / Justine J. Reel.
Description: Santa Barbara : ABC-CLIO, 2021. | Series: Q&a health guides |
    Includes bibliographical references and index.
Identifiers: LCCN 2021008316 (print) | LCCN 2021008317 (ebook) | ISBN
    9781440869891 (hardcover) | ISBN 9781440869907 (ebook)
Subjects: LCSH: Sexual harassment. | Sexual harassment—Psychological
    aspects.
Classification: LCC HQ1237 .R44 2021 (print) | LCC HQ1237 (ebook) | DDC
    305.42—dc23
LC record available at https://lccn.loc.gov/2021008316
LC ebook record available at https://lccn.loc.gov/2021008317

ISBN: 978-1-4408-6989-1 (print)
        978-1-4408-6990-7 (ebook)

25 24 23 22 21   1 2 3 4 5

This book is also available as an eBook.

Greenwood
An Imprint of ABC-CLIO, LLC

ABC-CLIO, LLC
147 Castilian Drive
Santa Barbara, California 93117
www.abc-clio.com

This book is printed on acid-free paper ∞

Manufactured in the United States of America

This book is dedicated to all "survivors" of sexual harassment. The #MeToo movement has given a voice to the many individuals who have suffered in silence for too long. My own realization that I had experienced sexual harassment as a college student during my coaching internship energized and prompted me to act and advocate. In my counseling practice, I have worked with many clients who have suffered silently from bullying and sexual harassment. I commit to give voice to victims of sexual harassment by speaking up and advocating for change.

Contents

Series Foreword

All of us have questions about our health. Is this normal? Should I be doing something differently? Whom should I talk to about my concerns? And our modern world is full of answers. Thanks to the Internet, there's a wealth of information at our fingertips, from forums where people can share their personal experiences to Wikipedia articles to the full text of medical studies. But finding the right information can be an intimidating and difficult task—some sources are written at too high a level, others have been oversimplified, while still others are heavily biased or simply inaccurate.

Q&A Health Guides address the needs of readers who want accurate, concise answers to their health questions, authored by reputable and objective experts, and written in clear and easy-to-understand language. This series focuses on the topics that matter most to young adult readers, including various aspects of physical and emotional well-being as well as other components of a healthy lifestyle. These guides will also serve as a valuable tool for parents, school counselors, and others who may need to answer teens' health questions.

All books in the series follow the same format to make finding information quick and easy. Each volume begins with an essay on health literacy and why it is so important when it comes to gathering and evaluating health information. Next, the top five myths and misconceptions that surround the topic are dispelled. The heart of each guide is a collection of questions and answers, organized thematically. A selection of five case studies provides real-world examples to illuminate key concepts. Rounding out each volume are a directory of resources, glossary, and index.

It is our hope that the books in this series will not only provide valuable information but will also help guide readers toward a lifetime of healthy decision making.

Acknowledgments

I would like to first acknowledge the detailed attention and patience of my developmental editor, Maxine Taylor. It is hard to believe that this book was written during a pandemic with schools essentially closed, but you continued to provide support to the project. My husband, Robert Bucciere, as always is my rock. Tackling a tough and emotionally intense topic like sexual harassment is not for the fainthearted. Having you at my side gives me the courage to face these types of societal challenges head-on. Amanda Tierney and Jenny Conviser—you are my female warriors and incredible collaborators on this important topic. You inspire me with your wisdom and partnership in bringing attention to these important issues in our field for those we serve. Maya Steel and Sonya SooHoo— thank you for your lifelong friendship and daily texts of encouragement. Finally, I have great appreciation for my parents who inspire intellectual curiosity and the importance of pursuing excellence.

Introduction

Have you ever felt that "spidey sense" of being uncomfortable when you are around certain people? Have you ever been on the receiving end of unwanted sexual advances at school or your place of employment? Has a teacher or supervisor abused their power by seeking sexual favors in return for good grades, positive reviews, or advancements? Maybe you have been in a situation where you were exposed to sexual banter or pornographic images. These varied examples represent sexual harassment.

Sexual harassment is defined as receiving attention of a sexual nature that is not desired or reciprocated. It can happen to anyone regardless of how they identify their gender or how old they are. Schools, places of employment, and being out in public can all serve as settings for sexual harassment to occur. Finally, although the stereotypical image of sexual harassment involves a male supervisor making unwanted advances toward a female subordinate, the harasser can identify as any gender.

When considering the forms that sexual harassment can take, it is important to realize that the types of sexual harassment may include verbal, physical, or cyber. Sexual harassment is often viewed as a form of bullying. Can you think of a time that you witnessed one of your classmates being called a derogatory name? That would be an example of verbal sexual harassment at your school. Physical sexual harassment could be characterized by unwanted touching or hugging among other displays of affection. Again, the key is that the behavior is not welcomed by the victim.

Cyberbullying is particularly dangerous as this form of sexual harassment takes place online typically using social media platforms. Comments of a sexually explicit nature can be posted, which are seen by many and continue well after the school day has ended. It is not hard to imagine that being exposed to these forms of sexual harassment and bullying would have a negative impact on the victim. Certainly, mental health suffers and results in increased depression, anxiety, and risk for suicide.

Sexual harassment is associated with other consequences as well, such as negatively impacting one's grades and academic career. If one is sexually harassed at work, the tendency may be to avoid the situation by missing work or quitting altogether. This can have a negative effect on one's likelihood of advancement and income. Therefore, the purpose of this book is to identify the ways that sexual harassment can be addressed. Steps that someone should take if they are sexually harassed are outlined, as well as the ways that a bystander or witness can intervene. Finally, specific ways that schools can confront sexual harassment and build a more accepting culture are discussed. It is our hope that this book will be a useful resource to teenagers, parents, community members, and other professionals. The question and answer format allows for easy navigation to find answers to the many topics within sexual harassment.

Guide to Health Literacy

On her 13th birthday, Samantha was diagnosed with type 2 diabetes. She consulted her mom and her aunt, both of whom also have type 2 diabetes, and decided to go with their strategy of managing diabetes by taking insulin. As a result of participating in an after-school program at her middle school that focused on health literacy, she learned that she can help manage the level of glucose in her bloodstream by counting her carbohydrate intake, following a diabetic diet, and exercising regularly. But, what exactly should she do? How does she keep track of her carbohydrate intake? What is a diabetic diet? How long should she exercise and what type of exercise should she do? Samantha is a visual learner, so she turned to her favorite source of media, YouTube, to answer these questions. She found videos from individuals around the world sharing their experiences and tips, doctors (or at least people who have "Dr." in their YouTube channel names), government agencies such as the National Institutes of Health, and even video clips from cat lovers who have cats with diabetes. With guidance from the librarian and the health and science teachers at her school, she assessed the credibility of the information in these videos and even compared their suggestions to some of the print resources that she was able to find at her school library. Now, she knows exactly how to count her carbohydrate level, how to prepare and follow a diabetic diet, and how much (and what) exercise is needed daily. She intends to share her findings with her mom and her aunt, and now she wants to create a chart that summarizes what she has learned that she can share with her doctor.

Samantha's experience is not unique. She represents a shift in our society; an individual no longer view themselves as a passive recipient of medical care but as an active mediator of their own health. However, in this era when any individual can post their opinions and experiences with a particular health condition online with just a few clicks or publish a memoir, it is vital that people know how to assess the credibility of health information. Gone are the days when "publishing" health information required intense vetting. The health information landscape is highly saturated, and people have innumerable sources where they can find information about practically any health topic. The sources (whether print, online, or a person) that an individual consults for health information are crucial because the accuracy and trustworthiness of the information can potentially affect their overall health. The ability to find, select, assess, and use health information constitutes a type of literacy—health literacy—that everyone must possess.

THE DEFINITION AND PHASES OF HEALTH LITERACY

One of the most popular definitions for health literacy comes from Ratzan and Parker (2000), who describe health literacy as "the degree to which individuals have the capacity to obtain, process, and understand basic health information and services needed to make appropriate health decisions." Recent research has extrapolated health literacy into health literacy bits, further shedding light on the multiple phases and literacy practices that are embedded within the multifaceted concept of health literacy. Although this research has focused primarily on online health information seeking, these health literacy bits are needed to successfully navigate both print and online sources. There are six phases of health information seeking: (1) Information Need Identification and Question Formulation, (2) Information Search, (3) Information Comprehension, (4) Information Assessment, (5) Information Management, and (6) Information Use.

The first phase is the *information need identification and question formulation phase*. In this phase, one needs to be able to develop and refine a range of questions to frame one's search and understand relevant health terms. In the second phase, *information search*, one has to possess appropriate searching skills, such as using proper keywords and correct spelling in search terms, especially when using search engines and databases. It is also crucial to understand how search engines work (i.e., how search results are derived, what the order of the search results means, how to use the snippets that are provided in the search results list to select websites, and how to determine which listings are ads on a search engine results page). One also has to limit reliance on surface characteristics, such as the design of a website or a book (a website or book that appears to have a lot of information or looks aesthetically pleasant does not necessarily mean it has good information) and language used (a website or book that utilizes jargon, the keywords that one used to conduct the search, or the word "information" does not necessarily indicate it will have good information). The next phase is *information comprehension*, whereby one needs to have the ability to read, comprehend, and recall the information (including textual, numerical, and visual content) one has located from the books and/or online resources.

To assess the credibility of health information (*information assessment* phase), one needs to be able to evaluate information for accuracy, evaluate how current the information is (e.g., when a website was last updated or when a book was published), and evaluate the creators of the source—for example, examine site sponsors or type of sites (.com, .gov, .edu, or .org) or the author of a book (practicing doctor, a celebrity doctor, a patient of a specific disease, etc.) to determine the believability of the person/organization providing the information. Such credibility perceptions tend to become generalized, so they must be frequently reexamined (e.g., the belief that a specific news agency always has credible health information needs continuous vetting). One also needs to evaluate the credibility of the medium (e.g., television, Internet, radio, social media, and book) and evaluate—not just accept without questioning—others' claims regarding the validity of a site, book, or other specific source of information. At this stage, one has to "make sense of information gathered from diverse sources by identifying misconceptions, main and supporting ideas, conflicting information, point of view, and biases" (American Association of School Librarians [AASL], 2009, p. 13) and conclude which sources/information are valid and accurate by using conscious strategies rather than simply using intuitive judgments or "rules of thumb." This phase is the most challenging segment of health information seeking and serves as a determinant of success (or lack thereof) in the information-seeking process. The following section on Sources of Health Information further explains this phase.

The fifth phase is *information management*, whereby one has to organize information that has been gathered in some manner to ensure easy retrieval and use in the future. The last phase is *information use*, in which one will synthesize information found across various resources, draw conclusions, and locate the answer to their original question and/or the content that fulfills the information need. This phase also often involves implementation, such as using the information to solve a health problem; make health-related decisions; identify and engage in behaviors that will help a person to avoid health risks; share the health information found with family members and friends who may benefit from it; and advocate more broadly for personal, family, or community health.

THE IMPORTANCE OF HEALTH LITERACY

The conception of health has moved from a passive view (someone is either well or ill) to one that is more active and process based (someone is working toward preventing or managing disease). Hence, the dominant focus has shifted from doctors and treatments to patients and prevention, resulting in the need to strengthen our ability and confidence (as patients and consumers of health care) to look for, assess, understand, manage, share, adapt, and use health-related information. An individual's health literacy level has been found to predict their health status better than age, race, educational attainment, employment status, and income level (National Network of Libraries of Medicine, 2013). Greater health literacy also enables individuals to better communicate with health care providers such as doctors, nutritionists, and therapists, as they can pose more relevant, informed, and useful questions to health care providers. Another added advantage of greater health literacy is better information-seeking skills, not only for health but also in other domains, such as completing assignments for school.

SOURCES OF HEALTH INFORMATION: THE GOOD, THE BAD, AND THE IN-BETWEEN

For generations, doctors, nurses, nutritionists, health coaches, and other health professionals have been the trusted sources of health information. Additionally, researchers have found that young adults, when they have health-related questions, typically turn to a family member who has had firsthand experience with a health condition because of their family member's close proximity and because of their past experience with, and trust in, this individual. Expertise should be a core consideration when consulting a person, website, or book for health information. The credentials and background of the person or author and conflicting interests of the author (and their organization) must be checked and validated to ensure the likely credibility of the health information they are conveying. While books often have implied credibility because of the peer-review process involved, self-publishing has challenged this credibility, so qualifications of book authors should also be verified. When it comes to health information, currency of the source must also be examined. When examining health information/studies presented, pay attention to the exhaustiveness of research methods utilized to offer recommendations or conclusions. Small and nondiverse sample size is often—but not always—an indication of reduced credibility. Studies that confuse correlation with causation is another potential issue to watch for. Information seekers must also pay attention to the sponsors of the research studies. For example, if a study is sponsored by manufacturers of drug Y and the study recommends that drug Y is the best treatment to manage or cure a disease, this may indicate a lack of objectivity on the part of the researchers.

The Internet is rapidly becoming one of the main sources of health information. Online forums, news agencies, personal blogs, social media sites, pharmacy sites, and celebrity "doctors" are all offering medical and health information targeted to various types of people in regard to all types of diseases and symptoms. There are professional journalists, citizen journalists, hoaxers, and people paid to write fake health news on various sites that may appear to have a legitimate domain name and may even have authors who claim to have professional credentials, such as an MD. All these sites *may* offer useful information or information that appears to be useful and relevant; however, much of the information may be debatable and may fall into gray areas that require readers to discern credibility, reliability, and biases.

While broad recognition and acceptance of certain media, institutions, and people often serve as the most popular determining factors to assess credibility of health information among young people, keep in mind that there are legitimate Internet sites, databases, and books that publish health information and serve as sources of health information for doctors, other health sites, and members of the public. For example, MedlinePlus (https://medlineplus.gov) has trusted sources on over 975 diseases and conditions and presents the information in easy-to-understand language.

The chart here presents factors to consider when assessing credibility of health information. However, keep in mind that these factors function only as a guide and require continuous updating to keep abreast with the changes in the landscape of health information, information sources, and technologies.

The chart can serve as a guide; however, approaching a librarian about how one can go about assessing the credibility of both print and online health information is far more effective than using generic checklist-type tools. While librarians are not health experts, they can apply and teach patrons strategies to determine the credibility of health information.

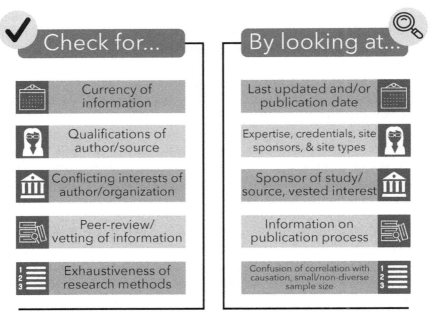

All images from flaticon.com

With the prevalence of fake sites and fake resources that appear to be legitimate, it is important to use the following health information assessment tips to verify health information that one has obtained (St. Jean et al., 2015, p. 151):

- **Don't assume you are right**: Even when you feel very sure about an answer, keep in mind that the answer may not be correct, and it is important to conduct (further) searches to validate the information.
- **Don't assume you are wrong**: You may actually have correct information, even if the information you encounter does not match—that is, you may be right and the resources that you have found may contain false information.
- **Take an open approach**: Maintain a critical stance by not including your preexisting beliefs as keywords (or letting them influence your choice of keywords) in a search, as this may influence what it is possible to find out.
- **Verify, verify, and verify**: Information found, especially on the Internet, needs to be validated, no matter how the information appears on the site (i.e., regardless of the appearance of the site or the quantity of information that is included).

Health literacy comes with experience navigating health information. Professional sources of health information, such as doctors, health care providers, and health databases, are still the best, but one also has the power to search for health information and then verify it by consulting with these trusted sources and by using the health information assessment tips and guide shared previously.

Mega Subramaniam, PhD
Associate Professor, College of Information Studies,
University of Maryland

REFERENCES AND FURTHER READING

American Association of School Librarians (AASL). (2009). *Standards for the 21st-century learner in action.* Chicago, IL: American Association of School Librarians.

Hilligoss, B., & Rieh, S.-Y. (2008). Developing a unifying framework of credibility assessment: Construct, heuristics, and interaction in context. *Information Processing & Management, 44*(4), 1467–1484.

Kuhlthau, C. C. (1988). Developing a model of the library search process: Cognitive and affective aspects. *Reference Quarterly, 28*(2), 232–242.

National Network of Libraries of Medicine (NNLM). (2013). Health literacy. Bethesda, MD: National Network of Libraries of Medicine. Retrieved from nnlm.gov/outreach/consumer/hlthlit.html

Ratzan, S. C., & Parker, R. M. (2000). Introduction. In C. R. Selden, M. Zorn, S. C. Ratzan, & R. M. Parker (Eds.), *National Library of Medicine current bibliographies in medicine: Health literacy.* NLM Pub. No. CBM 2000-1. Bethesda, MD: National Institutes of Health, U.S. Department of Health and Human Services.

St. Jean, B., Taylor, N. G., Kodama, C., & Subramaniam, M. (February 2017). Assessing the health information source perceptions of tweens using card-sorting exercises. *Journal of Information Science.* Retrieved from http://journals.sagepub.com/doi/abs/10.1177/0165551516687728

St. Jean, B., Subramaniam, M., Taylor, N. G., Follman, R., Kodama, C., & Casciotti, D. (2015). The influence of positive hypothesis testing on youths' online health-related information seeking. *New Library World, 116*(3/4), 136–154.

Subramaniam, M., St. Jean, B., Taylor, N. G., Kodama, C., Follman, R., & Casciotti, D. (2015). Bit by bit: Using design-based research to improve the health literacy of adolescents. *JMIR Research Protocols,*

4(2), paper e62. Retrieved from http://www.ncbi.nlm.nih.gov/pmc /articles/PMC4464334/

Valenza, J. (2016, November 26). Truth, truthiness, and triangulation: A news literacy toolkit for a "post-truth" world [Web log]. Retrieved from http://blogs.slj.com/neverendingsearch/2016/11/26/truth-truthiness -triangulation-and-the-librarian-way-a-news-literacy-toolkit-for-a -post-truth-world/

Common Misconceptions about Sexual Harassment

1. GIRLS OR WOMEN WHO DRESS OR ACT A PARTICULAR WAY ARE ASKING FOR SEXUAL HARASSMENT

One of the biggest barriers to tackling the problem of sexual harassment is an age-old assumption that girls and women somehow seek attention from others that is attributed to how they act or what they wear. Society's tendency to blame the victim sadly represents a common feature associated with violent crimes such as rape. This pattern of associating unwanted sexual advances to the victim's clothing or demeanor removes responsibility from the perpetrator. Thus, victims are dehumanized and often accused of "asking for it" by dressing or behaving a particular way (e.g., flirting or seeking the attention of the opposite sex). Individuals who are scantily dressed in clothing deemed inappropriate for school, such as low-cut tops, sexy skirts, or short shorts, may become targets of judgment and labeled as being part of the problem rather than viewed with compassion for the harassment endured. Despite this myth, sexual harassment can occur to anyone regardless of how a person dresses, and it should be underscored that they are not asking to be verbally harassed or receive other forms of sexual advances. If the recipient considers the attention to be undesirable, sexual harassment has occurred. Blaming a victim for their clothing choices or behavior undermines the severity of the act and is counterproductive for the fight against sexual harassment in workplaces and other settings.

2. ONLY GIRLS AND WOMEN ARE VICTIMS OF SEXUAL HARASSMENT; MEN CANNOT BE SEXUALLY HARASSED

It is often assumed that girls and women are the sole victims of sexual harassment. Although women report sexual harassment at a higher rate than their male counterparts, men and boys are victims of sexual harassment too. Furthermore, it is expected that many instances of male victimization go unreported. Bottom line is that sexual harassment can occur regardless of how a person self-identifies their gender identity. This means that a broader view should be taken when examining the complexities of sexual harassment to reach beyond the gender binary (male vs. female) and to extend to those who do not identify as man or woman. This narrow misperception that men do not face sexual harassment is often reinforced by traditional gender stereotypes and historical underpinnings of the original legislation designed to protect individuals against gender discrimination. Anyone regardless of their gender identity can be victims of unwanted attention of a sexual nature. Further, this myth falsely suggests that sexual harassment is about one's attraction to the opposite sex rather than a crime stemming from power and control tendencies of the perpetrator. People who commit sexual harassment are seeking power and will select targets perceived to be vulnerable to efforts of coercion. Male victims or individuals who do not identify as male or female may be victims of sexual harassment from a person in a position of authority who is of the same sex or of the opposite sex. The key is that the attention is of an unwanted sexual nature.

3. SEXUAL HARASSMENT IS MOTIVATED BY A DESIRE FOR SEX

Although sexual harassment may have some elements that resemble flirting or giving attention of a sexual nature that are present in a healthy romantic relationship, the myth that sexual harassment is motivated by one's sexual attraction needs to be dispelled. It is easy to attribute unwanted advances of a sexual nature, such as requests for sexual favors in exchange for a good grade or to gain special attention, to a physical or sexual attraction on the part of the perpetrator. Interestingly, sexual harassment is rarely about physical attraction to the victim. Much more frequently, these acts of sexual harassment are clearly tied to being dominant or asserting one's power over a subordinate, a younger person, or someone perceived to be vulnerable. The relationship between exerting control and committing sexual harassment is demonstrated by the tendency for vulnerable populations such as people with disabilities to be frequent targets of sexual harassment and bullying behavior at school.

4. HARASSMENT ALWAYS OCCURS BETWEEN A MAN AND A WOMAN; IN OTHER WORDS, THE PERPETRATOR OF SEXUAL HARASSMENT IS ALWAYS THE OPPOSITE SEX

This stereotype about sexual harassment is largely based on traditional gender roles espoused in older movies like *9 to 5*. In this popular film that was released in 1980, Dolly Parton plays the role of an administrative assistant to a sexist boss who breeds an environment at the workplace of gender discrimination and sexual harassment. Related to this stereotype is the common belief that sexual harassment involves a female victim who receives unwanted sexual attention from her male teacher, boss, older relative, or authority figure. It is important to note that sexual harassment can occur in any setting—workplace, school, or public places. Moreover, sexual harassment may take place between individuals of the same sex or of the opposite sex. In other words, it is quite possible that a male subordinate could be the victim of sexual harassment from a female supervisor—or a male one. A male student could be harassed by his male teacher. It is also important to reinforce that the perpetrator does not necessarily have hiring and firing authority and could be of equal status or rank within the organization. Finally, it is important to be inclusive to individuals who fall outside of the gender binary (trans) who may also be victims of sexual harassment. The key point is that the attention or behavior was unwelcome.

5. IF I REPORT SEXUAL HARASSMENT AT MY WORKPLACE, I WILL BE FIRED FROM MY JOB

Many employees (and some employers) feel powerless in making real and significant change in their workplace. It can seem as if the human resources department at one's office is protecting the company rather than the victim. To make matters worse, employees who have spoken up or issued a complaint and appear in the public eye have frequently been accused of reporting the incident to gain fame or fortune. With the high stakes of speaking up against the wrong things that are happening at the office, there is the perception that one faces a clear risk of losing one's job. Reporting something like sexual harassment to the authorities may be perceived as professional suicide. This leads too many employees to endure the bad behavior until they can leave the company rather than risking job loss. It is important to be realistic about the challenges associated with making a complaint, but that does not mean that a victim should not speak up. Although it takes a lot of courage to speak out against one's employer, supervisor, or colleague, if an employee does disclose sexual harassment in the workplace, they should be protected by law from retaliation associated with the formal complaint. In fact, the Equal Employment Opportunity Commission found that over three-fourths of victims (i.e., 87–94 percent) experiencing sexual harassment neglect to file a report. Most cases of sexual harassment go unreported for a variety of reasons. One problem is the fear that reporting sexual harassment will be even more uncomfortable or that one will be forced out of their position. But there are other reasons, such as denial, guilt, or shame, that can play a role in the decision not to report the unwanted attention.

QUESTIONS AND ANSWERS

QUESTIONS AND ANSWER

❖
Identifying Sexual Harassment

1. What is sexual harassment?

Sexual harassment as a concept is highly charged and often conjures up images of nasty courtroom battles or gender discrimination in the school or workplace. In short, sexual harassment is defined as any unwanted attention of a sexual nature that is offensive regardless of the person's intention behind the behavior. Sexual harassment can potentially occur in a variety of places such as at a restaurant, on the bus or playing field, social media, at a business, or even at church. Although the description of sexual harassment is seemingly well defined, identifying when and if sexual harassment has occurred can become more confusing when certain behaviors (e.g., joking in a sexual manner) are normalized in specific situations, peer groups, or settings.

What makes matters even more complicated is that some recipients will respond differently to the same type of attention than others. It is also possible that some individuals will perceive a certain behavior (or even the same comments) in various ways. In other words, within a school setting a male teacher could compliment two different female students about their fashionable outfits. That comment (whether innocent or not) from one's male teacher in this scenario could potentially yield two drastically different responses. One female student might view the attention from the individual as "making an effort" to bond with students and be

approachable whereas the other student might report feeling uncomfortable, awkward, or exposed. In the case of the female student who sees the
attention as undesirable or creepy, this situation could reflect or contribute to a culture of sexual harassment. It is also important to note that just
because a person is wearing revealing clothing, it does not make it acceptable for others to make suggestive comments or to provide unwanted
attention or criticism. It is good practice for teachers or persons in positions of authority to avoid making comments about a person's appearance
or clothing choices to prevent negative reactions.

Despite the clear evidence of inappropriate comments that are made
by persons of authority, it is often the recipient of such compliments, teasing, or verbal sexual harassment who are viewed in a negative light. The
myth that individuals who identify as women somehow provoke sexual
harassment due to wearing short skirts and tight clothing only perpetuates the tendency to blame the victim for the crime. When in doubt
about how comments regarding someone else's attire and clothing may be
interpreted (or experienced) by the target or recipient, it is always better
to refrain from making any comment at all, including one that may sound
complimentary in nature.

In contrast to other criminal acts, the intent of the person committing
the crime is not a factor for determining whether sexual harassment has
occurred. For murder, as an example, the law can result in different penalties being assigned based on whether the act is determined to be an accident or an act of self-defense or a self-meditated act. If a person is found
guilty of committing sexual harassment, however, the penalty is essentially the same regardless of the intention behind the behavior. Moreover,
it is also important to emphasize that harm is not always intended and
could involve a truly innocent remark or gesture. However, what is crit-
ically important when examining whether sexual harassment has taken
place is to consider the perception of the person at the receiving end of
the attention—whether it's a verbal comment, inappropriate touch, or
something else. Teasing may be done in a flirtatious manner, or it may be
perceived as bullying behavior, but the key question comes down to: "How
does the recipient of the teasing feel?" It is not uncommon for someone to
try to explain or defend bullying behavior or other shameful remarks (e.g.,
"you are eating well, aren't you?") by making light of them: "I was just
joking." If harm was caused and the person felt humiliated—it is bullying
rather than a poorly executed comedian routine.

In certain cultures, behaviors that have been historically normalized
in some groups might be immediately identified as improper and labeled
as sexual harassment. In the 1980s, women who worked on Wall Street

indicated that they did not call such behavior sexual harassment. They referred to it as "going to work." They knew receiving unwanted attention from male colleagues and clients came with the territory.

Situations can affect the context of the behavior or how it is perceived. For example, some sexual comments are intended as compliments and others are intended to be insulting. However, regardless of the environment one is in or the form it takes, sexual harassment is distinguished from flirting or other kinds of behavior or desired attention that involves interest being reciprocated. The key distinguishing feature in all cases is that sexual harassment (in the eyes of the victim) is seen as unwelcome and unwanted. In other words, this attention is undesirable, and if repeated, it often contributes to the existence of a hostile environment.

The challenge can be in nailing down how to identify what is not welcome for one person and can be considered nonthreatening and perfectly acceptable in another setting or by a different individual. There are certain signs that a behavior is unwelcome (and thereby sexual harassment) versus just fun and flirtatious. First, if the person (i.e., victim) is upset or clearly seems to be uncomfortable or embarrassed, the behavior is likely unwanted. Another way to view it objectively is to think about how you might respond if you received the same behavior; if you would feel upset, it is likely others could feel the same way. One caveat is that each person is different. A person's level of sensitivity, family history, previous experiences with the same and opposite sex, and the power dynamic of their role in an organization can all influence one's potential reaction to the same behavior. If the person who receives behavior does not reciprocate with similar behavior back, it was likely unwanted and unwelcome from the recipient's perspective.

As previously mentioned, unlike other types of criminal acts, the intent of the perpetrator is not meaningful in determining whether sexual harassment has occurred. Rather what matters here is the perceived impact of the behavior on the victim. In other words, just because someone does not mean to sexually harass an individual or make them feel uncomfortable, the perpetrator is not off the hook. How the attention is received and perceived by the target determines whether it is sexual harassment. Therefore, if an action is experienced as unwanted sexual attention, that is all that is needed to categorize it as sexual harassment. It goes without saying that certain forms of sexual harassment are obvious and clear cut when it comes to identifying that a violation has occurred. Unwanted touching or kissing are overt signs that sexual harassment has occurred. But how do people respond when they receive a compliment about their appearance such as a recent haircut or a new dress? It is natural for a person to react differently depending on the situation—at school, work, or a social situation like a party. It might also make a difference who delivered the compliment, don't you think? The relationship and rapport of the person receiving the comment do play a role in how well it will go over. Harassment can take on several different forms including verbal sexual harassment, cyber sexual harassment, and physical sexual harassment. Sexual harassment also fits into two broad categories: quid pro quo and hostile environment.

The verbal form of sexual harassment can involve a variety of behaviors. Engaging in sexually explicit talk or making sexual innuendos (e.g., references to sex throughout a conversation) can make others feel uncomfortable especially in an academic context like after-school activities, in the lab, or at one's internship. The stereotypic version of verbal sexual harassment might be cat calls or other shouting of an unwanted nature, like when a woman walks by a construction site or receives derogatory shouting from a passing car. It can be difficult to distinguish between sexual harassment and flirting because many inappropriate behaviors start to become accepted as the norm or couched as flattery (even by the adults who have the power to influence change). In fact, girls from a Minnesota study reported that boys often say bad things to them, but they have come to the realization that "boys will be boys" and they must get used to this type of treatment because there are usually minimal repercussions for their male classmates. Some common phrases female students report included the following: "Give me some booty," "Give me a lap dance," or "Looking good enough to eat." Female students often report peer-to-peer sexual harassment coming in the form of male classmates telling dirty and sexist jokes to them or in their presence.

Receiving comments from a classmate who is of the opposite sex about one's appearance might be an example as are more indirect references to sex or sexually explicit comments about others in the school. This can get tricky when the comments are conveyed in a teasing manner or are commonplace within one's friendship group. Furthermore, when a classmate repeatedly asks someone out on dates this can become inappropriate. In fact, this act can evolve into sexual harassment when the victim has continually said "no," and it can also fit the bill for verbal sexual harassment. Homophobic slurs or negative comments about one's sexual orientation represent yet another example of verbal sexual harassment. Studies have indicated that this type of sexual harassment is extremely common. Approximately 73 percent of female students had been called a lesbian, whereas 74 percent of male students had been "accused" of being gay. People who do not fit into the gender binary (identify as male or female), such as individuals who express themselves as trans often find themselves as targets of harassment, violence, and bullying.

People do not need to leave their homes to become exposed to either sexual harassment or bullying. An increasingly digital society has expanded the opportunities for harassing individuals outside of school and work. Smartphones and social media have opened the door for sexual harassment to occur round the clock and seven days of the week. Texts that are sexually explicit and involve unwanted sexual attention represent an example of cyber sexual harassment. Social media posts that are humiliating or embarrassing also can serve as ways for sexual harassment to occur. Examples of sexual harassment would also include posting photos or videos that portray the victim in a less than becoming light as well as making comments about someone's appearance. Although the history of cyber bullying is shorter than other forms of in-person bullying, it is clear that the impact can be irreparably damaging for the victim.

Physical forms of sexual harassment can include unwanted touching regardless of the intent. For example, a friendly classmate of the opposite sex decides to hug another student who then feels uncomfortable. This situation may be subtle and seem harmless compared to a supervisor who touches the legs of his female employees under the table during a business meeting against their will. Both scenarios could be considered examples of physical sexual harassment. Other examples of physical sexual harassment include, but are not limited to, flashing one's body or private parts, rubbing up against someone, or sitting too close to someone else. In school settings, physical sexual harassment is incredibly common and may become normative. Female students complain about sexual harassment behavior, including having their buttocks touched, grabbing of their private body parts, playful slapping, or having a classmate rub up against them. Another commonly cited behavior was having clothes pulled down. Almost all female students (91 percent) reported that they had experienced having their clothes pulled off. Over half of male students (59 percent) admitted that they had their clothes pulled down or off. Both male (55 percent) and female students (85 percent) reported being spied on while getting dressed or showering at school. As with other types of sexual harassment, the consistent theme across these behaviors is that the attention is unwelcome. Sexual harassment, regardless of the form it takes (verbal, cyber, or physical), has been formally categorized as quid pro quo and hostile environment harassment.

It is important to identify what type of sexual harassment has occurred or is happening. There are two broad categories of sexual harassment. The first type of sexual harassment is referred to as quid pro quo. Quid pro quo is the Latin phrase that literally translates as "something for some-thing." In other words, if I do this for you, you need to do this for me in return. This type of sexual harassment often refers to favors being given in exchange for the expectation that the favor be returned. Can you imagine if your teacher told you that you would get a good grade if you gave them a kiss? This scenario provides an example of quid pro quo sexual harass-ment. Another example would be if a swim coach told one of their swim-mers that they would be on the roster for the top heats during the next meet if they sent a picture of their private parts.

Although the quid pro quo type of sexual harassment can occur any-where, you probably most often think about this type of sexual harassment taking place in the workplace. There are many movies that have illus-trated a culture of sexual harassment and gender discrimination within the office. How is the workplace setting ripe for sexual harassment? First, people spend an enormous part of their daily lives at work. Their work network can begin to resemble a dysfunctional family. In addition, job security and opportunity for promotion often weigh heavily on the minds of workers. Quid pro quo can occur in the workplace when there is a clear power relationship between one's supervisor and the employee. If employ-ment decisions are based on requests of a sexual nature, sexual harassment of this type has taken place. For example, an employee receives negative scores on his annual review when he fails to accept his boss's invitation for cocktails after work. It is also possible for sexual harassment to take place among coworkers who do not have a clearly defined power dynamic. One employee could say, "I'll finish this project if you go on a date with me," which illustrates the offering of a favor in exchange for a favor type of sexual harassment.

In contrast to the quid pro quo type of sexual harassment that focuses heavily on the power dynamic between the perpetrator and victim is a second type of sexual harassment: hostile environment or hostile work environment. This type of sexual harassment can be much more difficult to prove than quid pro quo. Specifically, hostile environment represents a broader form of sexual harassment than quid pro quo and is based largely on the perceptions and experiences of the victim. For hostile environ-ment harassment to occur, the perpetrator's unwanted sexual advances contribute to an intimidating, offensive, or threatening environment for someone else (the victim). In this instance, the situation becomes increasingly more uncomfortable. Keep in mind that the hostile envi-ronment form of sexual harassment can occur in a variety of settings. Regardless of whether the sexual harassment occurs at work, school, or in a public place, the key factor is that a particular environment starts to feel toxic, extremely uncomfortable, or unbearable for the victim. Attributed to feeling uncomfortable at one's place of employment or school (i.e., experiencing hostile environment harassment), there is commonly an outcome of loss of productivity at work. This is unsurprising as the victim of the hostile environment experiences constant distractions associated with and in anticipation of further negative sexual conduct. It might be difficult to even walk in through the doors of one's workplace without having intensely negative or unpleasant feelings. To fit the bill for hostile environment, the actions in one's workplace or school must be unwelcome, sexual in nature, and repetitive. Unfortunately, this type of sexual harassment is more challenging to quantify and may persist for quite some time without being identified or resolved. In many cases, by the time the situation has been addressed the damage has already been done. It is understandable that the affected employee may feel compelled to leave their job to escape the sexual harassment and negative situation and start a new and more positive work chapter.

Experiencing the hostile environment type of harassment within the school setting can be particularly challenging. A student may not have the mobility or flexibility to change schools based on where one's family resides. Therefore, the victim may continue to be subjected to negative attention and may increasingly feel more uncomfortable. Unfortunately, this constant sexual harassment can lead to numerous negative health consequences.

Another aspect of hostile environment harassment is that the sexual conduct or behaviors might be normalized or considered commonplace in certain settings. There may be differing viewpoints, for example, if a conversation at lunch during the workday or school day becomes sexually explicit. While some of the participants may enjoy the discussion and actively contribute, others at the table may feel extremely uncomfortable. This potential for having divergent perspectives on the same issue creates ambiguity and sets up a situation that can potentially be riddled with misunderstandings. It is important that no person regardless of the setting or normative culture feel uncomfortable.

You might be wondering how flirting fits into the discussion of sexual harassment. The easiest way to delineate between sexual harassment and flirting is to think about the presence or lack of power between the two individuals. Flirting is considered harmless if both individuals are participating and there is equal participation in the social interaction, and no one is in control. In other words, harmless flirting exists when the playful banter is reciprocated and the relationship is egalitarian. For example, one person states, "That's a great dress." When the other person says,

"Why, thank you. You don't look too shabby yourself," the interaction is clearly friendly banter with no ill intent. However, if the person responds in a way that indicates they are clearly uncomfortable with the attention, that is a different story entirely. This dynamic morphs into sexual harassment when one person has power over the other such as if the person can make decisions that are harmful to the other person. Flirting should be discouraged by someone in an authority position like one's teacher or boss. To be on the safe side, it is wise to stay away from comments of a sexual nature or remarks that bring attention to on one's appearance. Going the conservative route for social interactions in the workplace or other settings is probably the best policy for preventing confusion whether you are a man or a woman.

2. What is the difference between sexual harassment, sexual assault, and sexual misconduct?

The purpose of this book is to answer common questions specifically about the topic of sexual harassment. However, the terms "sexual harassment," "sexual assault," and "sexual misconduct" are often used simultaneously. Therefore, it is important to note that there are distinct definitional and legal differences between each of these concepts. With a few exceptions, the responses to the outlined questions in this book focus primarily on sexual harassment.

Sexual harassment has been identified as any unwanted attention of a sexual nature in the workplace, school, or other settings (e.g., public places). Sexual harassment could occur in the form of verbal bullying or comments but can also encompass physical acts like touching. Sexual harassment behaviors that fall into the cyber category were described as harassment occurring online rather than in a face-to-face situation. For example, the use of social media to harass someone by posting negative comments or pictures would all fit the definition for sexual harassment.

Although a frequent occurrence, it is important to clearly state that sexual harassment is not legal. In fact, sexual harassment has been prohibited in the United States since the introduction of the Civil Rights Act in 1964. In other words, sexual harassment is covered by law and considered to be a form of gender discrimination. Sexual harassment is illegal (i.e., against the law) in professional settings, which means that in the workplace a penalty can be applied with unwelcome behavior regardless of the intention of the perpetrator. The quid pro quo (i.e., exchange of one favor for another) form of harassment could involve a person in a position of power making sexual demands from a subordinate in exchange for keeping one's job or receiving a promotion. Hostile work environment refers to sexual harassment that creates an uncomfortable work environment for the victim. This type of sexual harassment is viewed with respect to the severity of the behavior as well as frequency of behavior and whether the behavior would typically be perceived as offensive.

Although sexual harassment within a place of employment is illegal in every state, other behaviors that mimic sexual harassment outside of the professional setting are not necessarily punishable by law. For example, if a woman walks by a construction site and receives cat calls and whistles of an unwanted nature, this behavior is technically not against the federal law, even if it represents unwanted attention. However, certain states have gone the extra step to try to outlaw this type of behavior that can be perceived as threatening by the recipient. A significant challenge in our culture that should not be overlooked is that the victim of sexual harassment is often blamed for "asking for it" because of the way they dress or act. Until we stop blaming the victim, it will be difficult to identify and address sexual harassment in a direct manner.

In contrast to sexual harassment, sexual assault can represent a range of threatening or violent sex behaviors that are treated as criminal acts under both federal and state law. The United States Justice Department deems any behavior that involves sexual contact without explicit consent of the victim to be sexual assault. Examples of sexual assault include rape, forcible sexual contact of any kind, unwanted groping and fondling. The punishment for these behaviors varies from state to state. The type of behavior may also receive differing punishment. For example, groping as a crime is typically treated as a misdemeanor and is labeled as sexual battery. Under federal law, physical contact must be involved to be considered sexual assault. Therefore, comments of an unwanted sexual nature and exposing one's body parts would fit as sexual harassment rather than sexual assault. Perhaps you are familiar with the case of Hollywood media mogul, Harvey Weinstein, who famously brought public attention to sexual harassment and assault. There were numerous cases of sexual harassment and sexual assault brought up against him. He abused his power to force himself on young actresses in the context of a business arrangement and then swore them to secrecy. Certainly, the news of these cases once they broke out inspired the #MeToo movement and the eventual awareness about the pervasiveness of sexual assault in Hollywood and the workplace. Weinstein's behavior ranged from alleged rape to forcing someone to perform oral sex in his hotel room or office. Sexual abuse usually fits in this category as well if the victim is a minor (i.e., anyone under 18 years of age).

The term "sexual misconduct" is meant to be broad and is often used in the media to depict cases against celebrities and powerful men and women. Generally, sexual misconduct is not considered a legal term and does not refer to a specific criminal act or discriminatory behavior (such as gender discrimination through sexual harassment). The umbrella term can represent the spectrum of behaviors from requests for sexual favors within the workplace in exchange for promotion opportunities to teasing about a person about their appearance to groping. Similar to sexual harassment and sexual assault, sexual misconduct may be viewed and treated differently depending on the state laws. For example, groping is charged as criminal sexual conduct in Minnesota. Being charged with groping (e.g., touching a person's buttocks without consent whether over or under one's clothing) is punishable as a misdemeanor by Minnesota state law with a $3,000 fine and up to a year in jail.

3. Where can sexual harassment occur?

Sexual harassment can occur anywhere there are people. In fact, with the emergence of the internet and social media one can become a victim of sexual harassment without leaving their home. Although sexual harassment may be present in a variety of situations, the workplace is most frequently cited. It follows then that the origination of laws to prohibit gender discrimination is related to one's workplace sexual harassment. In addition, sexual harassment is frequently observed in school settings as well, such as kindergarten to twelfth grade and university campuses. Other situations where sexual harassment can occur include, but are not limited to, athletic teams, professional organizations, sororities and fraternities, military groups, home, online forums, and other public settings.

Perhaps when we picture sexual harassment in our mind, an image of a workplace comes to mind. For some of our readers who have seen the television show *Mad Men*, it is easy to think of examples of gender discrimination in the roles traditionally defined for women and men. The examination of the occurrence of unwanted attention of a sexual nature in the workplace demonstrates the many ways sexual harassment can have a nasty presence. The most obvious illustration of sexual harassment in a work setting is the abuse of power by a supervisor who bullies an employee into behavior that they does not want to engage in. Certainly, there are less overt ways that sexual harassment plays out, for example, by passing flirtatious remarks or by asking an employee out for a date (especially when it happens repeatedly after being turned down). Something as innocent as a comment about a colleague's appearance can even fit the category of sexual harassment if the remark is not desired by the recipient. Although the most stereotypical example of sexual harassment in the workplace involves a boss and employee, violations can also occur between persons of equal standing within the organization. It should also be emphasized that men can also be victims of sexual harassment. Furthermore, colleagues regardless of gender identity can commit sexual harassment or be victims of unwanted sexual attention.

It is alarming to learn that sexual harassment frequently occurs in both middle school and high school as well as on college campuses. Sexual harassment can happen between peers within the same grade or different grades. It is also possible for a teacher to abuse their power and engage in inappropriate behaviors such as making comments of a sexual nature toward a student. Alarmingly, more than 58 percent of female students reported experiencing sexual harassment from a school employee! It must be emphasized that although female students commonly fall prey to sexual harassment, male students can also be victims. Sometimes sexual harassment is tied to one's sexual orientation as well. Bullying behavior is often linked to sexual harassment within the school setting.

Sexual harassment within the school setting can include verbal comments or physical behaviors. Examples of verbal sexual harassment in school include making jokes or comments of a sexual nature, calling someone a homophobic name, making comments about the parts of someone's body, or asking someone out repeatedly despite being turned down. Another example would be making gender-demeaning comments or discussions of a sexually explicit nature in the presence of the victim as well as making threatening comments. Physical forms of sexual harassment could include pinching, touching or grabbing sexually, forceful kissing, brushing up against someone, or pulling one's clothing off. Other examples of sexual harassment in a school setting could be spreading sexual rumors, spying on someone who is showering in the locker room, writing sexually provocative messages on walls of bathrooms, displaying pornographic images, or cornering someone by standing too close. In the present day, bullying may also include using social media as a forum for posting comments of a sexual nature or those that discriminate upon the basis of one's sex or sexual identity.

College campuses can be a breeding ground for the occurrence of sexual harassment due to the many opportunities for social interactions that are both formal and informal. Sexual harassment may present itself in a variety of ways. In a clear abuse of power, a faculty member may abuse their power and make flirtatious comments toward a student. Another example of a faculty member exerting power is by expecting sexual favors in exchange for a strong grade in the course (i.e., quid pro quo sexual harassment). Sexual harassment may also occur in a campus dormitory where there is ample opportunity for students to mix and mingle during their down time outside of the academic setting. Two groups have been identified as high risk for a variety of negative behaviors including sexual harassment (and sexual assault): athletic teams and fraternities. Athletes are thought to represent the celebrities on campus, which brings a certain power along with it. Some athletes have abused this power and have exerted their "hero" status in a variety of ways that compromise the law. Although some of these ways may involve petty crimes such as property damage, other cases have involved blatant sexual harassment of other athletes—male or female—or students in the general population who are not members of athletic teams. This hubris or arrogance has sometimes been associated with cases of domestic violence, sexual assault, and rape. Similarly, fraternity groups have been identified as a breeding ground for sexual harassment and sexual assault. As part of hazing rituals for some fraternities, pledges were shown to be pushed to drink heavily while being encouraged to engage in a variety of questionable acts. Some of those behaviors involved sexual activity that was unwanted by male or female peers. Drinking alcoholic beverages has been shown to be related to sexual harassment and assault. Therefore, it follows that settings in which drinking is occurring (e.g., fraternity parties or college bars) might increase risk for such violations to take place. It should be underscored that being drunk or being tipsy does not give the perpetrator an excuse to engage in negative behaviors. In fact, one's ability to provide consent may be compromised if they have been drinking.

Unfortunately, a persistent stain for the military has been the multiple reports of sexual harassment. While cases of sexual harassment have not been limited to female military personnel, numerous women in the armed services have come forward with unfortunate stories that illustrate a pervasive disregard for sexual harassment. In some cases, the violations occurred repeatedly and out in the open without disciplinary action. Sexual harassment that has been reported in the military include unwanted comments or bullying that might be construed as flirtatious; however, many cases of blatant violations have been revealed. Women in the military who faced sexual harassment at all ranks reported being forced to provide sexual favors in exchange for advancement and promotions or be at risk of being singled out. Books like *Shoot Like a Girl: One Woman's Dramatic Fight in Afghanistan and on the Home Front* detail horrifying experiences of women in the military who face extensive sexual harassment. Mary Jennings Hegar of the Air National Guard and Air Force revealed a culture of constant discrimination based on one's sex, abuse of power, and risk of sexual assault throughout her time in the military. In addition to women who serve in the military, gay and trans individuals face higher risk of harassment.

As noted earlier, sexual harassment can happen anywhere and in the most unlikely times and places. Both men and women (as well as younger individuals) can become victims of sexual harassment while participating in extracurricular activities as well as more spontaneous forms of social interaction during unstructured time. Even going to a retail store or dinner party could present an opportunity for sexual harassment to occur. Sexual harassment may take place as a chance encounter or may be planned or recurring. Examples of sexual harassment include unwanted comments of a sexual nature by construction workers or inappropriate touching by a neighbor during a backyard picnic. Settings that tend to offer the opportunity for social interaction among strangers and acquaintances may lead to a familiarity that allows space for the occurrence of sexual harassment. Taking public transportation, for example, may lead to experiences that necessarily involve interacting with people outside of one's school or workplace. Having a predictable daily interaction could set the stage for sexual harassment. There has been much less attention placed on these types of settings than schools and the workplace even though public settings and community groups offer ample openings for both human interaction and sexual harassment.

While much of sexual harassment that is documented in cases throughout history involves face-to-face interactions, it is possible to be a victim by just going online. Children and adolescents growing up in the present generation can expect to witness or experience bullying at school and when they get home and are on social media. Social media offers the opportunity to interact with others and post comments, and with this comes the potential to become a victim of sexual harassment. For example, an "innocent" post on a friend's Instagram picture commenting on her appearance in a sexual manner might very well be unwanted and offensive. Dating sites, such as Tinder, Match, Bumble, and others that are driven by social media, also offer a ripe landscape for negative social interactions to occur, including sexual harassment. It is perhaps not surprising that providing this access to strangers might

create communication confusion, certain tensions, and misunderstandings. Online communication (e.g., emails and posts on forums) might be
misunderstood or may be more aggressive or direct than intended. There
is also a theory that people feel emboldened to say things online that they
would not have normally said in person. In fact, many individuals who
participate in online dating platforms report feeling uncomfortable with
the attention they are receiving from virtual strangers. Some individuals
report being stalked by individuals they have met online despite efforts to
move on to meet other contacts. There is increasing more evidence and
recognition of online avenues of sexual harassment, but much research is
needed in this area.

4. What are the warning signs that someone you know has been affected by sexual harassment?

Regardless of where sexual harassment takes places, many cases of sexual
harassment are never disclosed and reported. Therefore, to help reduce
sexual harassment and help victims when it has taken place, it is important to recognize the warning signs. The warning signs may differ depending on the age of the victim. For example, the symptoms may look one
way for young children and another way for adults who are victims of
sexual harassment. A noteworthy red flag is that children may talk in a
way that is "more adult" for their age (e.g., discussing topics of a sexual
nature) or may exhibit bedwetting. They may also avoid being alone with
certain adults. Children may also have nightmares or show excessive fear
or worry. Another potential warning sign related to sexual harassment is
noticing that an adult makes comments about the appearance (especially
of a sexual nature) of a child. If an adult is giving an unusual or excessive
amount of attention to a particular child or discussing adult topics with
them, it may also be a cause for concern.

Warning signs for teenagers may be similar to those red flags noted for
children. In addition, a teen who displays a lack of interest in self-care is a
cause for concern. For example, demonstrating poor hygiene by avoiding
showers (beyond what is typical for them) may be showing a sign of sexual
harassment or other problem. Other red flags include drinking or using
drugs, suicidal thoughts, self-harming behaviors such as cutting, or with-
drawing from normal behaviors. Another warning sign for a teenager is to
show a decline in one's academic performance, which may be exhibited
by failing grades or poor attendance.

Adults who are college students may also show a decrease in academic performance. College students may avoid certain classes or settings in which sexual harassment is taking place. In addition, college student adults may show emotional signs such as mood swings, low self-esteem, self-harm, and depression. Although college students have a unique social network in the academic environment, adults may face sexual harassment in the workplace. Generally, all adults regardless of age may show changes in mood, become withdrawn, or show drop in productivity. In the workplace, adults who are experiencing sexual harassment may be less likely to attend social events or avoid volunteering for projects. Moreover, if the adult is being harassed by their employer or supervisor, they may miss more workdays or take longer to complete projects.

It is critical to note that warning signs for sexual harassment may be of a physical, behavioral, or emotional nature. Many individuals will exhibit all types of warning signs, but most importantly, changes in one's behavior or emotional state are a telltale sign that there may be a problem.

Emotional warning signs include mood swings as well as symptoms of depression, anxiety, panic attacks, or post-traumatic stress disorder. Although mental health issues can be hard to detect, when a person demonstrates a significant change in mood that is different from what they typically display, that is the time to take notice. Is your friend at school more jumpy than usual? Do they appear sad or stressed out or exhibit feelings of hopelessness?

Examples of behavioral signs are talking excessively about sex or dressing provocatively. Covering up or disguising one's body is also a potential behavior that could represent a warning sign for sexual harassment. A person who is experiencing sexual harassment may also avoid being alone or in the same room as one's perpetrator and attending social events or may miss classes or work. If the perpetrator is in one's family, the victim may isolate oneself during family functions or avoid going altogether. Do you notice if a coworker is missing work functions or certain meetings when they have regularly attended in the past? This could be a sign that there is a problem.

Physical signs may include, but are not limited to, complaining about headaches and stomachaches, evidence of fatigue, increased stress, or sleep disorders. Inability to sleep is a common problem related to sexual harassment. Individuals may oversleep after experiencing sleep difficulties. This tendency may impact being punctual for work, school, or family functions. A person may show a change in hygiene as evidenced by messy or unkempt appearance. The existence of eating disturbances, such as eating too much (e.g., emotional eating or binge eating episodes) or eating too little, can also represent red flags for sexual harassment. Associated with eating disturbances a victim of sexual harassment may exhibit weight gain or extreme weight loss.

5. How prevalent is sexual harassment in the United States?

The prevalence of sexual harassment is difficult to estimate for numerous reasons. Firstly, to be included in the national prevalence data, the incident must be reported. There is often shame or fear of misunderstanding that can prevent sexual harassment from being reported. In addition, there can be fear of the potential consequences associated with being a whistleblower such as losing one's job. Silence is a common feature of sexual harassment. According to reports from U.S. Equal Employment Opportunity Commission (EEOC), 70 percent of women who have experienced sexual harassment at their jobs fail to report the incident to prevent negative repercussions of a personal or professional nature. For instance, Hart Research Associates conducted a 2016 survey and estimated that 40 percent of girls and women who work within the fast-food industry and occupied jobs that were not at management level experienced sexual harassment in the work setting. This included behavior such as jokes or teasing of a sexual nature, unwanted kissing, or suggestions about one's sexual orientation. Unfortunately, 42 percent of these girls and women expressed that accepting sexual harassment as part of the job was necessary to retain their position (even if at a fast-food establishment). It is important to note that even if these girls or women can afford to lose their jobs, they are unlikely to have the means to engage in the legal fight necessary to battle sexual harassment they have experienced. If they choose to report the incident to human resources, many girls and women (and male victims) express experiencing retaliation in the workplace or school setting, which is extremely unbearable. This fear of retaliation often leads those who do report to do so much later and after they have already left their place of employment.

Despite these barriers to achieving an accurate count, the overall prevalence of sexual harassment has been estimated to be 81 percent for women and less than half (43 percent) of men. It is expected that boys and men who report sexual harassment may experience stigma and therefore are less likely to identify being a victim of sexual harassment. When looking at locations where sexual harassment had occurred, it should be noted that 69 percent of women and over a quarter (or 26 percent) of men reported sexual harassment in public spaces. Alarmingly, one does not need to leave one's home to experience sexual harassment as 37 percent of women and 18 percent of men reported sexual harassment online. Women reported sexual harassment at a higher rate (i.e., 38 percent) than their male counterparts (i.e., 13 percent) in the workplace. In addition to women showing significantly higher rates of sexual harassment, certain groups of people are thought to be more vulnerable and thus at higher risk for sexual harassment. Examples of vulnerable groups include individuals with disabilities, people who serve in the military, and the adolescent population.

One group, individuals with disabilities, represents a vulnerable population who may be more likely to experience sexual harassment. In one study, 69 percent of women with disabilities were found to experience physically aggressive sexual harassment, whereas fewer women who did not have disabilities (59 percent) reported experiencing physically aggressive sexual harassment. For sexual assault, the numbers were more alarming. Forty percent of women with disabilities reported sexual assault compared with 23 percent of women who did not have disabilities. By contrast, 18 percent of men with disabilities experienced sexual harassment versus just 4 percent of men who did not have disabilities.

People who serve in the military have also been identified as a population at higher risk for experiencing sexual harassment. It has been acknowledged by many sources that incidents of sexual harassment and assault are widely underreported; however, anecdotal evidence has revealed compelling stories of mistreatment and abuse of service members. The current prevalence numbers within the military are as follows: 22 percent of women reported sexual harassment (in general) with only 7 percent of men in the service admitting to being sexually harassed. When getting specific about the type of sexual harassment, it was found that 21 percent of women and 7 percent of men in the military reported experiencing a hostile work environment. For the quid pro quo type of sexual harassment, the prevalence dropped to nearly 2 percent of women and less than 1 percent of men in the military. Once again, the secretive nature of this problem should be emphasized, which means that underreporting has likely occurred, and thus, prevalence rates are viewed with caution. Recently, female legislators Claire McCaskill and Kirsten Gillibrand have focused on sexual harassment. They have pointed out that true estimates have been difficult to predict because the military is largely shielded from sexual harassment complaints that do not see the light of day. Unfortunately, when claims occurred, it was found that there was a strong likelihood that retaliation and power would occur. Only two in ten would report incidents. Of the women who did report sexual harassment in the military, approximately 62 percent felt that they experienced retaliation following their claim. In a 2014 study, the Department of Defense Sexual Assault Prevention and Response deployed a survey about sexual harassment and found that 116,600 service members reported being sexually harassment, which equated to around 22 percent of female participants and 7 percent of male participants.

Unfortunately, like the military, schools can serve as a breeding ground for sexual harassment. Teenagers in the United States most likely face some type of unwanted attention. This negative attention very possibly takes the form of sexual harassment at school. In fact, four of five teens (i.e., 81 percent) reported experiencing some type of sexual harassment in school according to a study conducted by the American Association of University Women. As anticipated, more girls than boys experienced sexual harassment in schools. Specifically, most of the girls (i.e., 85 percent) and over three-fourth of boys (76 percent) reported sexual harassment. However, the frequency of sexual harassment is most notable when considering the gender. Almost one in three girls (31 percent) selected "often" as the response to frequency of experiencing unwanted advances compared to only 18 percent of boys. Sexual harassment usually begins in middle school or junior high (grades sixth through ninth). Nearly half of female and male students were harassed during middle school. For girls, 54 percent reported experiencing sexual harassment compared with 40 percent of boys. Alarmingly, one in three of those students (32 percent) had experienced harassment prior to seventh grade. Thirty-four percent of girls and 32 percent of boys had received sexual harassment before entering seventh grade. Another study reported lower prevalence estimates when taking into account school-age children ranging from pre-K to twelfth grade. In this case, almost one-third of female students (or 30 percent) and 14 percent of male students had experienced some form of sexual harassment.

When breaking down the incidence of sexual harassment by behavior, the statistics may be even more startling. Almost all female students (92 percent) and over half of male students (54 percent) experienced being forced to do something sexual (other than kissing). Nearly 90 percent of female students and 63 percent of male students had been subjected to sexual rumors. Over half of female students were pressured to do a sexual act against their will, and a quarter of all students reported experiencing unwanted touching. With regard to frequency, over half of female students (57 percent) and 21 percent of male students complained of feeling harassed every other day or once per week. Most of these acts represented peer-to-peer sexual harassment (89 percent).

6. How is sexual harassment viewed in countries around the globe?

Although the United States did not really touch the issue of sex discrimination in the workplace until 1964 and that eventually extended to include sexual harassment, it was still ahead of other countries around the globe. Sexual harassment and how it is perceived is largely driven by the cultural norms in one's country. For countries that tend to uphold traditional gender roles and stereotypes (e.g., women are less important than men), there is a greater likelihood that sexual harassment will be normalized or even accepted. This tendency to largely take sexual harassment for granted was pervasive in the previous decades for the United States despite the strong stance the #MeToo movement has taken against sexual harassment in recent years. Interestingly, sexual harassment in the workplace is considered illegal by most jurisdictions around the world. South Africa as an example refers to harassment as an unfavorable treatment or degrading behavior based on sex. There may not necessarily be an element of sexual desire for harassment to have occurred and could include insults, threats, or nonverbal behavior that somehow ties to a barrier in achieving gender equity in the workplace. Although laws have existed, there has been a paucity of research on this topic (including in South Africa), and actual statistics of sexual harassment offenses often fail to be available to show the prevalence of a problem within the country.

While the United States has brought the issue of sexual harassment back into the spotlight with the #MeToo movement and subsequent Time's Up movement, other countries have also been fiercely committed to the development, revision, and enforcement of law to protect individuals against sexual harassment in the workplace and beyond. For example, Great Britain, Canada, and Australia hold similar interpretations in their law by interpreting sexual harassment as a type of sex discrimination. Although the label appears the same, there have been vast differences in how cases of sexual harassment are handled within these countries and across the globe. Interestingly, one study showed that of the 23 countries that were surveyed, only seven countries actually had statutes that recognized or identified the concept of sexual harassment, and the law seemed to be applied unevenly.

For some countries, such as Australia and Canada, statutes against sexual harassment applied at the federal level and the state or province level. For other countries, the statute took place at the state level including Sweden, Spain, New Zealand, France, and the United States. To complicate matters, some countries, such as Australia, Canada, Switzerland, United Kingdom, and Ireland, mentioned sexual harassment in statutes and then further defined the term by using judicial decisions. Another interesting consideration when looking at the phenomenon of sexual harassment around the globe is who is protected by the laws. There has largely been an assumption that sexual harassment is a problem that primarily afflicts women. Thus, this assumption has meant that other groups have not been afforded the opportunity for protection under the law. Although there have been some similarities across countries, each individual country represents a slightly different view and implementation of sexual harassment.

Regardless of whether formal laws are in place and regularly enforced, the interplay between cultural norms of what is "right" and "wrong" behavior when it comes to sexual misconduct cannot be ignored. For example, in Scandinavian countries such as Sweden where gender equality is widely promoted through employment and family life, sexual harassment is frowned upon and employers are expected to prevent and address them. In 2016, the Swedish government tightened legislation to penalize workplace discrimination. To take it a step further, the Swedish Work Authority was provided instructions in 2018 from the government that they (i.e., the Authority) should conduct business in a way that promotes a workplace that values diversity and gender equality. Moreover, the place of employment should be free from both discrimination for any reason or risk for victimization. In Swedish schools, government funding has been provided to the Children's Welfare Foundation to distribute materials to create awareness about sexual harassment in primary and secondary schools. Starting these initiatives early is thought to give clear expectations for appropriate and inappropriate behaviors when it comes to gender interactions.

In 2018, a new law change in Sweden makes it mandatory to have explicit consent between partners for any sex act for it not to be considered rape. This included cases where the person did not actively say "no." While this consent is required for current law around sexual assault, the difference is that this law change introduces the categories of "negligent rape" and "negligent sexual abuse." These "negligent rape" charges can be brought when sexual assault was not intended by the perpetrator, nor was there violence associated with the act. One year later after the implementation of this law, human rights organizations claim it has had an impact on convicting cases of rape, and it visibly shows a tougher stance on sexual assault.

Although countries like Sweden have a reputation for gender equality and protecting the rights of women, that is not necessarily the case in other parts of the world. In Saudi Arabia, for instance, gender differences have been stark, traditional roles, and sexual assault and harassment have historically been overlooked or gone unpunished, or in worst cases, the female victim has been persecuted for the crimes committed against her. In groundbreaking legislation in 2018, Saudi Arabia passed laws to combat sexual harassment and reduce fear among women for living a normal life. Sexual harassment in Saudi Arabia has been defined as words or actions that hint at sexuality of another person, undermine the modesty of another person in any way, or harm another person. While technically illegal, like other countries, sexual harassment has gone largely unreported. In fact, there are no current sexual harassment statistics to report as a baseline. This new law is aimed to protect all human beings regardless of gender. The law also applies across settings such as school, workplace, orphanages, homes, and social media. The strictest penalties will be for actions taken again the vulnerable—such as children under 18 years of age and those with disabilities. Most severe cases will receive up to five years in prison and/or a monetary penalty (equivalent to $80,000).

Saudi Arabia has taken additional measures to improve the quality of life and position of women in society. The Kingdom has demonstrated some strong reforms with the Vision 2030 targeting ways to decrease the segregation of the genders and to have women more involved than ever before. An example of this is that women are eligible to drive cars now. It is important for cultural norms to slowly shift if sexual harassment laws have the necessary teeth to address and prevent these acts from taking place.

7. What are the laws against sexual harassment in the United States?

Sexual harassment is against the law, plain and simple. A broad legislation was passed in the United States at the federal level to protect against gender discrimination called the Title IX of the Education Amendments of 1972. For federally funded institutions whether, public or private entities, there is the requirement to follow Title IX. In schools, this law attempts to prevent any discrimination on the basis of one's sex. Further, this law protects both male and female students from experiencing sexual harassment within the United States by upholding this law from several decades ago.

When considering the historical context of sexual harassment, the life span is somewhat surprisingly short. Specifically, sex discrimination was not determined to be illegal until 1964 when a member of the Congress proposed an amendment to that which would in effect consider sex discrimination illegal along with race discrimination. Ironically, this amendment was proposed as an attempt to block a bill (that outlawing race discrimination) from passing; however, the bill did become law, and the amendment to outlaw sex discrimination was kept intact. Congress ultimately passed the Equal Employment Opportunity Act, which gave power to the Equal Employment Opportunity Commission (EEOC) eight years later in 1972. President Nixon signed the Education Amendments (i.e., Title IX), which effectively meant sex discrimination was illegal for any educational program in receipt of federal funding. The EEOC guidelines were eventually established and published under the leadership of Chairwoman Eleanor Holmes Norton more than 15 years after Title VII was passed.

Having this set of guidelines encouraged the public to recognize sexual harassment as a form of sex discrimination and encouraged employers to take positive steps against it. However, the history of sexual harassment laws has not been straightforward, and another setback was experienced when the transition committee for the Reagan Administration recommended that the EEOC guidelines be pulled back. In 1981, the U.S. Senate held hearings, chaired by Utah's long-standing senator, Orrin G. Hatch, regarding the nature of EEOC guidelines and whether they were considered antibusiness. Fortunately, despite these challenges, the EEOC guidelines survived the crossfire and were upheld. However, victims continued to face an uphill battle when reporting sexual harassment and dealing with discrimination in court. For example, in 1986 a female victim who brought a suit against a hospital in St. Louis for sexual harassment was not supported. The medical sales representative claimed that she experienced sexual harassment by a male supervisor who played a pornographic movie called *Deep Throat* at a work meeting. The four-million-dollar lawsuit brought by the employee Olivia Young was denied by a Missouri court.

The early cases of sexual harassment were not ruled in favor of victims in the early 1970s. For example, in the *Corne v. Bausch & Lomb* case, harassment by a supervisor was reported by two women who worked for a manufacturer of eye care products in Arizona. The case was not held up in court, and the employer was not held responsible for the reported sexual harassment. In another case, the Justice Department was charged with sexual harassment that resulted in the lower court awarding the victim $16,000 in damages. However, the Justice Department appealed and won the case. The victim, Diane Williams, who refused sexual advances from her supervisor, was fired nine days later from the Justice Department. In a third case, *Mill v. Bank of America*, the court ruled in favor of the employer. The reported sexual harassment was deemed an "isolated misconduct," and the employer was not held responsible. However, in 1979, this ruling was reversed by the Ninth Circuit.

In the academic context, sexual harassment was documented under Title IX of Educational Amendments in a case brought forward in 1977. Specifically, an undergraduate student at Yale University reported that her professor sought sexual favors in exchange for a better grade in the course. When the student refused to act on his unwanted sexual advances, she received a "C" instead of the "A" promised in the course. This led not only this female student but also four other students and a faculty member to file sexual harassment claims. In *Alexander v. Yale*, the sexual harassment case against the professor was dismissed.

Until the groundbreaking *Barnes v. Costle* sexual harassment case, the cards seemed stacked against the victims. However, in 1977 the U.S. Court of Appeals for the District of Columbia ruled in favor of a female victim who reported that that she was terminated from her government job when she refused to submit to her supervisor's sexual advances. The court determined that the case represented illegal sex discrimination and that if the employee had not been a woman she would not have been treated this way or lost her job. Therefore, this case set the important precedent for upholding the law against supervisory misbehavior.

Fortunately, there have already been laws in place that protect people in the United States from sexual harassment and other forms of discrimination. Although sexual harassment was recognized as a public concern starting in the 1970s, major federal laws had been in place even before it was recognized and labeled a societal problem. The major challenge to eliminating sexual harassment in the United States has always been an unwillingness on the part of the victim to report the crime and a culture that supports the continued discriminatory behavior against girls and women. When victims have reported instances of sexual harassment, they have not always been adequately protected and in some cases have been vilified or have faced retaliation in the workplace. Whistleblowers are not usually in the best position for job promotions.

In order to provide the necessary legislation to address this issue, Title VII of the Civil Rights Act came into existence in 1964, but it has been used to protect the rights of people in present day against problems such as discrimination including sexual harassment. Other notable federal laws include Title IX of the Educational Amendments of 1972. Title IX is often associated with sports and continues to be much debated as to whether it helped or hindered women's sports. However, Title IX goes much beyond sports in public institutions like high schools and college campuses. In fact, sexual harassment has become a pivotal issue within academic settings, and public institutions have a legal obligation to act and protect students. To this end, universities regularly hold mandatory training seminars on Title IX to raise awareness among academic leaders, faculty, staff, and college students about their responsibility if they become aware of sexual harassment.

The bottom line is that educational institutions have a legal obligation to protect individuals from sexual harassment on campus as well as for programs that are educational in nature and held off campus (e.g., student organization socials, course internships). Further, both quid pro quo and hostile work environment types of sexual harassment must be prohibited according to federal statutes and regulations.

8. What does consent mean?

There is often some confusion around the role of consent related to sexual harassment. It further muddies the water that laws about consent vary from state to state. There is also variation across situations from a legal perspective. How is consent given and what does it mean? At the crux of the matter is that there is a level of respect and trust that is the foundation of consent. Consent is defined as the agreement between two human beings to engage in activity of a sexual nature. In other words, there is a clear intention that is made known by both people that sex is desired. By contrast, there is no denying that engaging in activity of a sexual nature without obtaining consent is punishable as sexual assault or rape.

It is important to note that consent for a certain behavior is not a blanket agreement to continue that sexual activity. For example, if you have kissed someone in the past you have not given that individual permission to kiss you again in the future. In other words, consent must be given every time. Although it is not required, verbal communication to give consent is helpful. Communication is key to setting healthy boundaries in all relationships.

Another aspect of consent is that a person has the right to change their mind at any time. Although this might be frustrating for the other individual, they must respect the wishes of the person giving consent. If you find yourself in a situation where you no longer wish to engage in a certain behavior, it is necessary to state your change of heart. Saying something like "I know we have done X (fill in the blank) in the past, but I no longer wish to do this" is a clear and direct way to set boundaries and withdraw consent.

When seeking or providing consent to engage in a particular behavior, it is equally important to avoid ambiguity. A way to solicit consent might be to say, "Are you comfortable with this?" or "Is this okay?" If giving positive consent, a person should respond in the affirmative. If a person says "no" or wriggles away, it is critical for the other person to respect the physical or verbal cues that denote obvious feelings of being uncomfortable.

Other areas to consider when determining consent include age and alcohol or drug use. Specifically, laws are in place to protect minors (usually under the age of 18) from being encouraged to engage in sexual activity with someone older than them. A person who is underage for one's state or country cannot give consent for the behavior. If an adult has sexual activity with a person who is underage, they are committing a crime. They will be registered as a sex offender and likely will go to jail. Likewise, a person who is incapacitated due to abuse of alcohol or other substances cannot offer consent. It should be emphasized that one's appearance such as dressing in a provocative manner cannot be associated with consent. Moreover, if a person has previously engaged in a certain behavior that does not guarantee that consent has been provided across all situations. As underscored above, consent must be offered each time and must contain the following components represented in the acronym of "FRIES."

In order to provide education about the key elements of consent, the Planned Parenthood created an acronym (i.e., FRIES) to depict what to remember. The "F" in FRIES stands for "freely given" and underscores that providing consent is always a choice. Making this decision should not be done under the influence of substances such as illicit drugs or alcohol. No one should feel pressured or manipulated to consent to unwanted activity of a sexual nature. The "R" represents "reversible" and underscores the point that people have the right to change their minds. This right applies even if the two individuals have engaged in sexual activity in the past or are in the middle of a make-out session. Although uncomfortable and awkward, it is better to stop a situation at any point if it is not wanted. The "I" refers to "informed." Being informed means that both people are making the decision with all of the information available to them. Are both partners engaging in mutually monogamous sex? Is birth control being used by either partner? Do the rules change in the middle? The "E" stands for "enthusiastic." It goes without saying that both people should be excited or should want to engage in activity. No person should feel forced into something they do not desire or be with someone they don't care for in that way. Finally, the "S" is characterizing the need to be "specific." As mentioned throughout this response, consent should be given for each activity or behavior (e.g., kiss) every time. There is no such thing as blanket consent.

9. When were the first sexual harassment cases documented?

Sadly, the practice of sexual harassment has been around for many centuries even before sexual harassment had a name. Historians refer to slavery within the United States to illustrate examples of African American women who were slaves and early victims of sexual harassment and sexual assault at the hands of their owners. Perhaps surprising is that discrimination on the basis of one's sex has been illegal in the United States only since 1964. The Civil Rights Act was designed to eliminate employment discrimination based on one's race, sex, religion, or national origin and was the formal way of demonstrating that legal recourse could be taken against sexual harassment in places like the workplace. This law was dubbed "Title VII" in order to reference the portion of the law that covers an employment context. Interestingly, Title VII was broad enough to cover both gender discrimination of women and men; however, the primary intent initially was to target discrimination that women faced in the workplace. In 1972, this prohibition of discrimination was expanded to educational settings.

Title IX (commonly recognized for promoting gender equality in sports) was instituted to ban discrimination based on one's sex in schools that are recipients of federal funding. It was noteworthy that the Equal Employment Opportunity Commission (EEOC) determined that sexual harassment represents a form of discrimination by sex covered by Title VII. As noted, the law against discrimination for one's sex was passed in the early 1960s. There were several cases that have been documented in the 1970s that are related to sexual harassment. For example, the *Barnes v. Train* case from 1974 has often been labeled the first sexual harassment case in the United States. Paradoxically, the words "sexual harassment" were never used in this case, which was later dismissed. Specifically, Paulette Barnes, a payroll clerk who worked for the Environmental Protection Agency (EPA), complained that her male supervisor had made sexual advances toward her. When those unwanted advances were not reciprocated, she claimed that she lost her job. Although the case was initially dismissed, it was successful appealed. In the 1977 *Barnes v. Costle* case, Ms. Barnes won when the District of Columbia Court of Appeals determined that losing one's job after refusing to give sexual favors to one's male supervisor was indicative of sex discrimination. This case, although less prominent than the pinnacle 1986 case, was important in that the court ruled that companies are responsible if they are aware of sexual harassment occurring in the workplace and can be held liable. Although the words "sexual harassment" were purported to have not been uttered in the 1974 case, there is evidence that activists from Cornell University can be credited with coining the term "sexual harassment" in 1975. Another case in the 1970s was the *Williams v. Saxbe* case. This case argued that quid pro quo sexual harassment fits the definition of discrimination for one's sex under the Civil Rights Act. In this case, Diane Williams revealed that she lost her job when she refused to have sex with her male supervisor. This case was able to set the stage for future lawsuits for quid pro quo sexual harassment.

Although these 1970s' cases were important, sexual harassment cases did not receive any significant attention or real traction until the 1980s. It is suspected that the lack of attention to these cases as well as the reason more cases were not brought forward in the late 1960s and 1970s was more of a product of culture rather than lack of sexual harassment occurring in the workplaces at the time. In other words, receiving sexual harassment (or unwanted sexual attention) was sadly seen as "part of the job" by many female employees during that time period. Not only was this negative and inappropriate behavior expected, but it was also normalized within the work environment. Unfortunately, sexual harassment was so commonplace and pervasive that the behavior was not seen as illegal or something worth bringing forward in the form of a grievance. Luckily, attitudes began to shift over this time, and eventually, there was some movement in the courts system related to sexual harassment.

In the 1980s, the Supreme Court began hearing cases, and there were pinnacle cases during the decade that set the foundation for what continues to be a difficult legal battle. The case that is often pointed to as the "first" one to be recognized as specifically sexual harassment as a violation of Title VII was a U.S. labor law case of *Meritor Savings Bank v. Vinson*. Michelle Vinson was employed as a teller for the Capitol City Federal Savings and Loan Association in Washington, D. C. At the bank, Vinson faced repeated instances of sexual harassment from her supervisor for three years within the workplace. Vinson indicated that enduring this recurring sexual harassment led to a hostile work environment and therefore was a violation of the Civil Rights Act of 1964. The Supreme Court ruled in a 9-0 decision that sexual harassment is a form of sexual discrimination. Further, sexual harassment is strictly prohibited by Title VII. This first

case represents a landmark decision for sexual harassment and recognizes
this violation of the Civil Rights Act from 1964 as being actionable by
the law. Employers took notice and became more aware of sexual harassment. Additionally, the cases for sexual harassment grew exponentially,
signaling that a cultural shift was underway. Suddenly, sexual harassment
was an issue to be taken seriously by employers who realized that they
could be held liable.

One very public case with historical relevance is the 1991 Anita Hill
case that received much media attention due to the political stakes associated with the case. A law professor, Anita Hill argued that she had experienced sexual harassment under the direction of Supreme Court justice
nominee Clarence Thomas. Although the senate confirmed Thomas's
nomination, the public nature of the case brought much-needed awareness to the issue of sexual harassment. Moreover, the Civil Rights Act was
amended in 1991 to allow for a jury trial in seeking damages of compen-
satory and punitive nature for violations of Title VII. Both evolutions are
said to influence the increase of sexual harassment cases from 1991 (6,127
cases) to 1996 (15,342 cases). It is noteworthy that under federal laws
victims could receive more significant awards resulting from employers
and companies being held liable.

10. What are common characteristics of a harasser?

Much attention has been paid to the characteristics of the victim of sexual harassment. In some cases, the victim is wrongly accused of being
promiscuous, drinking too much, or dressing in a way that invites sexual
harassment. Unfortunately, this focus on tearing apart the victim does not
help the cause of raising awareness or addressing the broader issues surrounding sexual harassment. Thus, it is important to also learn more about
the perpetrator to hopefully develop some insight into sexual harassment.

This section focuses on whether there are any common characteristics
for individuals who are accused of sexual harassment. Developing a profile of certain features that are typical across perpetrators could serve as
red flags or help with early training and prevention. While the focus of
this section is to identify any patterns, it is also important to emphasize
that perpetrators can be of any age, sex, body type, race, or ethnicity. It is
equally critical to recognize that the context of harassment matters. Having a context that passively allows comments of a discriminatory nature
to go unchecked would contribute to a "culture" that is likely to be social-
ized to be more accepting of sexual harassment. For example, making

gendered references to "he" or "man" rather than making the swap out with a gender-neutral statement of "they" or "person" can represent the presence of implicit gender bias. Certain workplaces have more tolerance for gender bias and sexual harassment, but it is also necessary to consider the individuals who interact with others in their environment.

Ultimately, it is impossible to tell if someone will become or is a perpetrator of sexual harassment by looking at them. People who commit sexual harassment can come from any economic background and may come from an intact family or single parent household. There is no "magic formula" for what makes a perpetrator; however, there are some predictors as well as some myths that are not supported by research.

A common stereotype is that people who sexually harass identify as men. In fact, most people think of male bosses when they conjure a sexual harassment scenario, whereas both men and women can harass their coworkers, supervisors, or subordinates. Moreover, a harasser may be of any gender identity and could be married, in a relationship, or completely single. With respect to race and ethnicity, the harasser may self-identify as Black, white, Hispanic, Asian, or fill in the "other" category. The harasser may be straight, gay, or bisexual. Despite the fact, that anyone, regardless of their race, gender, age, or other characteristic can be a harasser, there are several factors that may be associated with people who are doing the harassing.

Firstly, people who are sexual harassers act when the opportunity strikes. They seek ways they can put others down to make themselves feel better. This predator mentality means that they observe (or stalk) their target prior to acting. When they do act and harass, it will usually be in a place where there are no witnesses and they are alone with their victim. Unfortunately, these circumstances mean that it is the victim's word against the harasser in the common "he said, she said" bind.

Another common characteristic of harassers is denial. It is common for harassers to blatantly refuse to view their actions as inappropriate or illegal. They may even wonder why their attention is not appreciated or seen as flattery. Harassers tend to be out of touch with reality and do not pick up on social cues.

The role of power and control cannot be overstated for the harasser. In a separate entry, it is a myth that actions to give a person unwelcome sexual attention are about having a romantic or sexual attraction first and foremost. In fact, these behaviors stem from wanting to exert power, keep the target in their place, and maintain control. For example, bringing up a woman's appearance or sexuality is a way to keep her off balance and uncomfortable in school or in the workplace. These individuals are extremely insecure and exhibit low levels of self-esteem. Bullying and committing sexual harassment is a way to make these harassers feel empowered and better about themselves.

It should be noted that alcohol has been identified as a common trigger for sexual violence across research studies. Although alcohol may increase risk for sexual harassment to take place, there are also circumstances such as in the workplace in which unwanted sexual attention occurs devoid of drinking. It should also be emphasized that a harasser is not necessarily a sex-crazed human being. In other words, the acts of sexually harassing one's peer in school or colleague are not usually motivated by wanting sex but rather by exerting power and control. Some research has shown that offenders tend to express a lack of empathy, have the inability to see clear boundaries, or may have been victims of childhood abuse themselves.

Interestingly, four psychological profile categories of individuals who harass others have been described by psychologist Dr. Ellen Hendriksen. The first category has been referred to as "the dark triad," and the individuals exhibit psychological characteristics of narcissism, psychopathy, and Machiavellianism. Being narcissistic means that the perpetrator is overly consumed within themselves. They display a lack of empathy and cannot understand the views of others. Narcissists feel they deserve to have power and be placed on a pedestal—people often describe them as having a big ego, being self-centered, and showing a lot of arrogance.

Psychopathy is associated with being manipulative, aggressive, and impulsive. They pretend to be empathetic but only for the purposes of exploiting victims into complying. If the opportunity presents itself to a psychopath, they will sexually harass. Finally, Machiavellianism refers to being deceptive and acting without morals. A person who displays Machiavellianism will do anything to achieve their goals regardless of the cost to others.

The second profile category refers to having the psychological characteristic of moral disengagement. Unfortunately, in this case, rules do not apply to the harasser because they have created their own version of reality that includes a separate set of rules that inevitably justify one's behavior. Sexual harassment is seen as acceptable and even desired by the victim. The perpetrator may see the event as a sexual affair rather than an unequal power dynamic associated with unwanted sexual attention. With this moral disengagement, the perpetrator has a tendency to blame the victim and show dehumanization. This perpetrator may point to the dress attire of the victim or that she was alone and out late. This psychological tendency allows the perpetrator to discount any moral compass or societal norms of right or wrong.

Another characteristic associated with the perpetrators is the tendency to work in traditionally male-dominated fields. For example, the type of employment could be a clue as jobs that are thought of as more masculine seemed to come with higher rates of sexual harassment. Examples include the police force, finance, entertainment, medicine and surgery, high tech jobs, and the military. Other jobs would include blue-collar employment in factories, construction, and mining that are considered to be male-dominated occupations.

Having a hostile attitude toward women is another predictor of sexual harassment. Not only are women viewed in traditional and stereotypical ways but also women are seen negatively. These strongly negative attitudes toward women can lead to the creation of a hostile climate or workplace.

Social scientists have attempted to classify the personality characteristics of harassers in the interests of better understanding who is more likely to be a perpetrator. One such study identified several types of men who were more likely to sexually harass others. The first type of men was represented by individuals who demonstrated extreme naïveté about relationships with the opposite sex. These men have been labeled misperceiving harassers. The second type of harassing men comprised individuals who tend to exploit their relationships with others, especially women (i.e., exploitative harassers). The third type comprised men who held strong negative feelings for women and were dubbed misogynistic harassers. Although there is evidence that women also can engage in sexual harassment behaviors, gender stereotypes lead us to the assumption that women and girls are victims of male perpetrators who harass them. However, in the 2020 book titled *#MeToo in the Corporate World: Power, Privilege, and the Path Forward*, a chapter is devoted to "women as predators," and cases have emerged over the years of female teachers harassing and victimizing their male students. Likewise, women can harass other women. In fact, 13 percent of women indicate that sexual harassment occurred by another woman. Some of the initial findings indicate that abuse of power is a key feature regardless of the gender of the perpetrator. For example, a male student's dissertation advisor who happens to be a woman can determine his fate and whether he graduates with his doctorate degree. If the sexual advances are not reciprocated, there is the potential for hurt feelings and, worse yet, retaliation with dire consequences. There is also the potential for women to harass other women. Although men are more often the victims of sexual misconduct by women, it is possible to have female-on-female sexual aggression.

11. What are workplace romances?

The issue of sexual harassment can be muddied by the presence of dating relationships in any context. With respect to jobs, the trend of more women entering the workplace has been associated with more opportunity to meet members of the opposite sex. This accessibility of human interaction and to get to know others on a deeper level has led to the somewhat natural tendency to develop romantic attractions. Patterns have emerged to indicate that approximately 33 percent of romantic relationships originate and possibly take place within the work setting. Dating in the workplace is highly controversial and can present many complications; however, research suggests that, workers who participated in a romantic relationship in their workplace reported some positive outcomes. For example, participation in such a relationship tended to relate to higher job satisfaction, increased involvement with work activities, improved intrinsic motivation, and better morale of both parties.

Unfortunately, there are numerous problems with having workplace romances. A perception problem can exist for other employees within the workplace regarding questions around whether a bias exists that may lead to one colleague being favored over another. Moreover, the presence of a workplace romance can be distracting for the parties involved as well as their coworkers. Many romantic relationships have ups and downs, and colleagues may feel pulled into dysfunctional interpersonal dynamics and experience pressure to take sides. Some studies have found that workers report concerns that overall productivity could be compromised when workplace romances occur.

An additional layer of complexity arises when romantic relationships that occur in the office are dissolved. Hurt feelings can impact the overall mood and morale in the office. Both parties must continue to interact and work together on projects. At the extreme, workplace romances can elevate the risk for complaints of sexual harassment (especially when the supervisor is in a relationship with a subordinate). Unfortunately, unwanted sexual attention can happen once the romantic relationship has ended, which can lead to sexual harassment lawsuits. Further complications can emerge if there is a perception of retaliation on part of one employee toward the other.

Ultimately, the general rule is that personal relationships are private and should not affect one's work productivity. Although the supervisor may feel little power to intervene, one aspect that is nonnegotiable is the conflict of interest inherent in a supervisory relationship. Regardless of whether a couple is dating or married, one's supervisor should be reassigned to avoid perceptions of impropriety.

Unsurprisingly, one study found that when workers were found to be in unequal roles the relationship was viewed as less appropriate than if colleagues were of an equal status. If a person in the workplace romance was married, the negative perception was even greater. Furthermore, if a woman was married but engaging in an adulterous workplace romance, she was viewed more harshly than men who were committing adultery of this nature. The gender of coworkers also has an influence on one's tendency to approve of workplace romances. Women were more likely to display negative attitudes toward workplace romances than their male counterparts. Paradoxically, women themselves were more likely to report having been involved in a romantic relationship at the office. Assumptions around motives for workplace romances also varied by gender. Men were labeled as engaging in office romances to boost their ego and for selfish reasons. By contrast, women were assumed to be motivated by emotion (e.g., love) rather than power or ego. Interestingly, of the women who admitted being in workplace romances 13 percent reported that their primary reason was the pursuit of job goals.

Consensual romantic relationships in the workplace are not without challenges. It is widely acknowledged that in our busy society it can be difficult to meet people, and it is not uncommon to have sexual attraction to a colleague who is likeable and has many positive qualities. Some of these relationships will represent employees who date their superiors, which can represent a power imbalance within the workplace. In fact, one recent study cited in the 2020 book called *#MeToo in the Corporate World: Power, Privilege, and the Path Forward* indicated that 11 percent of employees knew about a colleague who had a sexual relationship with a boss or supervisor. The majority (71 percent) of employees felt that sexual relationships with one's supervisor or boss were inappropriate for the workplace. Unfortunately, even when these relationships are mutual, having workplace romances can create unfair power dynamics and can disrupt the office culture and morale. In fact, employees reported a toxic work environment due to the following reasons associated with these office romances: 1) decreased morale—approximately one-quarter of employees felt that dedication and commitment was reduced; 2) respect was compromised for both the boss and the subordinate; and 3) productivity could take a hit as the team performance decreased.

Causes and Risk Factors

12. Why does sexual harassment occur?

Sexual harassment is certainly a complex issue, and therefore, no simple explanations exist for why it occurs. However, many researchers who study sexual harassment have focused on the power dynamics in society for some answers. In other words, theories for sexual harassment tend to argue that sexual harassment is related to an attempt to gain power. Several models exist to show why sexual harassment occurs in the United States and around the world. These theories include the natural or biological model, the organizational model, and the sociocultural model.

First, the natural or biological model claims that human beings have a natural attraction to the opposite sex, which drives them to seek sexual relationships. This model also argues that men have higher sexual drives than women, which results in a greater likelihood of males acting aggressively in a sexual manner. Clearly there are numerous problems with this possible explanation and theory. Researchers have expressed concerns that such assertions could imply that sexual harassment is somehow natural or expected.

Another theoretical explanation is referred to as the organizational model. The organizational model theory attributes the source of sexual harassment to the power inherent within organizational structures. In other words, having hierarchies within the workplace creates power dynamics that create an environment ripe for sexual harassment.

A third theory related to sexual harassment is referred to as the socio-cultural model. This model looks to dynamics related to social categories within the society that contribute to stereotypes and one's vulnerability to experience discrimination. The sociocultural model acknowledges that people experience treatment based on the color of their skin, gender, or other social characteristics. Moreover, this model can offer some connections between a patriarchal society and the existence of norms that enable sexual harassment behaviors to continue unnoticed or unchecked in many cases. Although none of these models have received widespread support, they all seem to suggest that power is at play with respect to sexual harassment. While power can help explain many cases of sexual harassment (e.g., those that involve a subordinate and one's supervisor), these theories cannot address cases that involve colleagues of the same position or cases wherein a subordinate employee abuses a supervisor. Much more research is needed to expand the theoretical base of this field of study.

13. Do both males and females experience sexual harassment?

The focus of many media stories has been girls and women who experience sexual harassment, but in fact, yes, both males and females, as well as individuals who identify outside of the gender binary, can be the victims of sexual harassment. This tendency to place a disparate amount of attention on cases that involve females as victims has played out for a variety of reasons. The data suggests that the incidence rates for women reporting sexual harassment are much higher than those of their male counterparts. Certainly, this gender disparity likely reflects a variety of factors but does not allow us to fully grasp differences in the way men and women are sexually harassed. Sexual harassment in general has gone unreported and underreported. For men, the likelihood of reporting is even lower in certain studies, but this finding related to gender has been mixed. There has been a paucity of research on men as victims of sexual harassment, but several studies are underway to better understand the relationship dynamics in which harassment occurs, as well as the psychological mindset of the harasser.

When considering the workplace as a potential setting for sexual harassment, research has suggested that there are gender differences in attitudes or perceptions of the severity of sexual harassment. Specifically, women and men view a variety of factors related to sexual harassment differently. Women are seen to view sexual harassment as a bigger issue, and gender differences have been reported with respect to how one feels about being sexually harassed at work. For example, men who are sexually harassed are significantly more likely to indicate feeling flattered than their female counterparts. In a 2005 study that examined the influence of gender and age on sexual harassment, researchers found that women were more likely to avoid reporting sexual harassment, which contradicted previous findings. Reasons cited for the lack of reporting included fearing that nothing would be done to address and resolve the situation and end sexual harassment as well as fearing retaliation. In addition, some female employees reported having the knowledge of no action being taken in other cases of sexual harassment at the workplace. This unfortunate circumstance has been underscored by the Harvey Weinstein scandal. Numerous victims have come out since the original allegations, showing the broad reach of his sexual harassment and assault in the workplace.

Female employees were much more likely to be knowledgeable about one's organizational policies and procedures around sexual harassment. They also reported feeling victimized resulting from their experiences with sexual harassment more often than their male counterparts. The intersection of gender and age was important when considering the appropriateness of behaviors in the workplace. Older women were significantly more likely to indicate that developing personal relationships in the workplace was unacceptable and inappropriate than the younger female employees. Furthermore, older women seemed to think that men might leverage their sexual attractiveness to get ahead and receive promotions (which was an interesting take). Older male employees reported being less likely to experience hostile work environment form of sexual harassment than younger male employees. Older men also possessed strong knowledge of organizational policies and procedures around sexual harassment and seemed to know coworkers who had experienced sexual harassment.

Another important distinction to make between women and men is how they define sexual harassment. In earlier studies, it was found that women tended to label more behaviors as sexual harassment than their male colleagues. Behaviors that were overlooked by men or felt was a gray area of sexual harassment were seen as sexual harassment by women. Women reported receiving compliments about their appearance, casual stares, or comments about one's body as unwelcome attention, which thus met the definition for sexual harassment. More recent work has uncovered that perceptions about what counts as sexual harassment have evened out and that fewer gender differences exist in the workplace. It was noteworthy that over 80 percent of male and female employees felt that receiving sexual remarks about one's body or clothing denoted sexual harassment. More than 90 percent of employees regardless of gender reported that pressure to go on a date or engage in sexual activity that was unwanted constituted sexual harassment. Finally, more than 70 percent of male and female coworkers agreed that language of a sexual nature and/or unwanted staring fell within the definition of sexual harassment. Over half of male and female respondents indicated that the following behaviors also met the definition of sexual harassment: making jokes of a sexual nature, making excessive eye contact, touching the other person, and having pinups in one's office space. It is promising to see increased agreement between the genders about what constitutes sexual harassment in the workplace although much work remains to be done to educate both employees and supervisors.

Women are slowly rising to positions of authority and supervising both male and female employees. However, the trend toward people in roles of authority committing sexual harassment has not translated into women in leadership roles being perpetrators disproportionately like we see for men in power positions. Several theories and explanations have been identified to help us comprehend what is happening with this gender-based phenomenon.

One explanation that is not fully supported due to lack of available data argues that research demonstrates that women have traditionally been less likely to initiate sexual relationships with direct reports, supervisors, or colleagues. On examining traditional gender roles, it was found women were less likely to "make the moves" on men and instead dropped hints, but there could be a cultural shift well underway. Dating apps offer the opportunity for both sexes to take the lead in asking out a potential date.

Another plausible explanation is that men simply do not view themselves as victims of sexual harassment even when the behavior has occurred. This tendency could be related to that men do not feel threatened or that their safety is compromised. Interestingly, some men reported feeling flattered rather than intimidated by sexual advances of their female colleagues. This response is likely linked to deeply embedded gender roles and how girls and boys continue to be socialized in subtle but different ways from inception.

A third explanation is that women have not traditionally held powerful positions that possess the necessary authority to undermine a male's career if he does not provide the expected sexual favors (i.e., quid pro quo sexual harassment). This explanation is becoming outdated as more women are rising to leadership roles within organizations.

Finally, men may not realize they can be victims of sexual harassment. When considering cases of gender discrimination and sexual harassment, the cases that have been highly publicized mainly have involved women as targets. Boys and men who have not received the necessary training to fully understand sexual harassment may not even realize that a violation has occurred. A male victim's response (like many female victims) may be embarrassment and humiliation. Men who have been sexual harassed by someone of the same sex may fear that being a target might be viewed in a negative way. These unwanted sexual advances are perceived as threats to their masculinity. This tendency toward homophobia or fear of being viewed or accused of being gay may further prevent a male victim from coming forward to report the incident. In fact, research has suggested that sexual harassment against men that had occurred within the same sex had more severe and pervasive consequences than when harassment had happened with the opposite sex.

The purpose of one study in the late 1990s was to assess attitudes toward sexual harassment of men by harassers of the same or opposite sex. The researchers had participants answer questions about several scenarios as potential jurors. They were asked to review cases of sexual harassment against men occurring within the same sex or the opposite sex. The cases judged most harshly were those involving the same sex. These incidents (i.e., sexual harassment against men involving same sex) were perceived to be more inappropriate, serious, and offensive than those wherein females were harassers in the fictitious examples. Furthermore, those cases received the harshest penalties and higher monetary damages and were more likely to receive guilty verdicts in the study. These results were consistent regardless of how the participant answered a list of questions regarding homophobic attitudes.

In considering overall incidence rates by gender, sexual harassment cases reported by women as victims clearly outnumber those of men. Interestingly, male victims of sexual harassment more often report being the target of same sex sexual harassment than sexual harassment involving the opposite sex. Therefore, regardless of the victim's gender, the consistent variable has been men as the identified harasser.

As indicated earlier in the section, not much data exists around male victims. However, some patterns have emerged for both male and female victims of sexual harassment. In addition to having a male harasser, the most common behavior involves sexual teasing and jokes. The second most common behavior for men (and women) relates to receiving unwanted invitations for dates and phone calls or messages. The challenges of studying sexual harassment of men include having measures that are modified to address the experience of men. Like eating disorder measures that were originally geared toward understand how women and girls experienced negative body image and disordered eating, sexual harassment survey questions need to reflect gender norms and experiences of male victims. It is also important to expand the discussion beyond the gender binary to include trans individuals and those who do not identify with a particular category.

14. Are certain groups of people more likely to experience sexual harassment than others?

Certain groups and social contexts are more prone to sexual harassment. As discussed in Question #12, women have consistently reported a higher tendency to experience sexual harassment than their male counterparts. Although there is some complexity with respect to reporting when it comes to boys and men, females have been identified as an "at risk" group for this negative behavior whether it be in a school setting, the workplace, or in public. Other considerations such as race and ethnicity, age, and disabilities have been identified to increase a person's vulnerability to becoming the target of sexual harassment; however, it should be reiterated that no one is immune to this negative behavior.

Girls and women may be a target for a perfect stranger or may experience sexual harassment from a supervisor or coworker. Traditional gender roles that place males in position of authority and power and women in subservient roles persist. The more male dominated a particular workplace is, the higher likelihood that sexual harassment will occur. Examples would include work sites that are typically considered more oriented toward this masculine identity such as manual labor (e.g., construction, landscaping, factory work). Moreover, the military has rich traditions and is baked in masculinity themes. Women who serve in the military are increasing in overall numbers, however, sadly reports of sexual harassment and assault are rampant. Many of these cases come to surface once the person has completed their service or left the military. Efforts have been made to contain the cases of sexual harassment within the military community to avoid tainting the image of the military, but it is evident that the military represents another group that is vulnerable to sexual harassment.

In addition to gender as a factor that may lead to increased risk for sexual harassment, the intersection of race/ethnicity should also be considered. Some studies have found that women of color are at additional risk due to being both female and a person of color. Specifically, Black and Latina women were found to experience comments and behavior consistent with sexual harassment associated with a culture of hypermasculinity. This culture of "machismo" for Latina women meant that she could be a victim of sexual racism—that is, experience discrimination for her race and her gender. This tendency carried over to Black women who reported being the target of derogatory comments at school, the workplace, and public. Comments seemed to come through a racist filter but were also sexist (and at times sexual) in nature. Sexual harassment was perceived as a way to put the victim in her place or to prevent her from getting promoted, gaining confidence, or being successful.

Some statistics have suggested that age is a risk factor for sexual harassment. Teenagers, for example, may find themselves in more situations where bullying and/or sexual harassment is likely. Middle school and high school can be hot beds for unwanted teasing. There is also some evidence that older adults may be at risk for sexual harassment. Due to increased vulnerability, senior citizens have been identified as victims of many types of abuse. It is a challenge because they may have issues with memory impairment, hearing loss, or visual impairment that may impede their ability to be fully in charge of their life decisions and be protected against discrimination or negative behaviors from others. Sadly, in many instances the harasser is a family member or home health worker—the very people this older adult depends on each day. It is important to prevent elder abuse as this group represents a large segment of our aging population within the United States.

Individuals with physical and intellectual disabilities are also at increased risk to experience sexual harassment. These individuals may be perceived as naive and may be easy targets for harassers who are seeking power and convenience. Not only are these individuals often socially isolated within their communities, but also if they do report sexual harassment, they are not always taken seriously. Individuals with intellectual disabilities may not have the ability to communicate coherently what happened and may not have the resources or support to press charges. As individuals are mainstreamed in public school systems, there is an increased potential for them to be the target of both sexual harassment and bullying in certain classrooms.

While ableism represents discrimination against individuals with disabilities, it is also important to consider the motivations of heterosexism and transphobia for acts of hate and sexual harassment. Heterosexism refers to discriminatory acts against individuals due to their sexual orientation or gender identity. Specifically, an at-risk group for bullying and sexual harassment includes individuals who self-identify as LBGTQ (stands for Lesbian Bisexual Gay Trans Queer) community. Sexual harassment may occur in school settings, places of employment, or public places (e.g., night clubs). Negative behavior may include derogatory comments or unwanted sexual advances that fit in the sexual harassment category, but it may also escalate to include sexual assault and physical violence. More information will be provided with respect to gender identity and sexual orientation in the next question.

15. What do gender identity and sexual orientation have to do with sexual harassment?

There has been some confusion and inconsistency surrounding whether gender identity and sexual orientation are considered a protected class and the enforcement of associated discriminatory acts within the workplace. Thankfully, U.S. Equal Employment Opportunity Commission (EEOC) offers the same protection for gender identity and sexual orientation as other protected classes (e.g., sex, age, race, national origin, religion, disability) under Title VII's prohibition of gender discrimination within the employment. Specifically, the EEOC interprets and enforces Title VII to protect LBGT employees even when there are contradictory state or local laws that do not offer such protection against discrimination.

Examples of forms of discrimination related to gender identity or sexual orientation include failing to hire an employee due to their sexual orientation or if someone identifies as a transgender. An employer cannot fire an employee due to gender transition or their sexual orientation. Another example of discrimination relates to offering equal access to restrooms. Much has been in the news about the North Carolina bathroom bills. Employees must have equal access to a restroom that represents their gender identity to avoid discrimination claims. Failing to promote someone due to sexual orientation whether gay or straight also represents discrimination. An individual who is paid a lower salary because of their sexual orientation or health insurance benefits are denied to one's spouse who is of same sex represents discrimination. Finally, harassing an employee due to sexual orientation or gender identity such as making derogatory comments is a clear example of employment discrimination.

The definition of sexual harassment (i.e., behavior that is unwanted sexual attention) remains the same regardless of the victim's sexual identity. Although stereotypes surrounding workplace sexual harassment often conjure a male supervisor as the harasser and the female subordinate as the victim, there are many possible scenarios that could play out. A female lesbian boss could just as likely be the harasser, and there could be gender discrimination that occurs within individuals who identify as of the same sex.

Research that focuses on sexual harassment has generally lacked diverse samples and neglects to expand beyond traditional gender roles of man and woman or heterosexist assumptions. In order to fully understand the extent and impact of sexual harassment, studies need to include individuals who identify as transgender or transsexual as well as to understand sexual harassment that occurs within same-sex relationships. As emphasized throughout this book, no one is immune from sexual harassment. Its close cousin of bullying strongly suggests that members of the LBGTQ (i.e., lesbian, bisexual, gay, trans, queer) community might be easy targets for individuals looking to exert power in places of employment, schools, and other public venues. Moreover, there are numerous examples in which LBGTQ individuals have been bullied online and over social media forums.

In fact, just as women have become targets of sexual harassment, one's sexual orientation (i.e., identifying as gay, lesbian, bisexual, trans, etc.) may put someone at increased risk of becoming a victim. Even those being perceived as the "other" (e.g., men who are suspected of being gay) were found to be at higher risk of becoming a target for sexual harassment. Women who identified as lesbian also reported increased risk of sexual harassment and assault that were tied to homophobic slurs and behaviors. On a college campus survey conducted at Yale, researchers discovered that a lesbian student was not only threatened with rape but was also called names like "dyke" and was the target of unwanted attention by a group of male college students.

Examples like the above underscore that there is an additional layer of discrimination that goes beyond gender when one considers the intersection of sexual orientation. While university students, faculty, and staff generally responded in accepting the ways of gay and lesbian individuals on campus, victimization rates were high for individuals who did not identify as heterosexual. Behavior that was both sexist and homophobic included the tendency of making stereotypical comments about gay, lesbian, or bisexual individuals. Graffiti contained language and symbols that were sexist and homophobic. Individuals who were considered the "other" due to sexual orientation were ostracized and alienated socially. They were made to feel alone, which resulted in increased risk for depression, self-harming, and suicide. These individuals also faced accusations that they were "gay" or "lesbian" as well as received threats to reveal their identity to others (e.g., students, family, friends). In some cases, these victims were forced to conceal or reveal their sexual orientation against their will.

Harassment experienced with respect to one's sexual orientation represented both violent acts (e.g., sexual assault) and verbal comments. Because of the secretive nature of sexual identity, many cases of sexual harassment go unreported. There is a fear of being "outed" during the police investigation of the crime or once someone has reported sexual harassment at work or school. Moreover, lesbian women anticipate negative attitudes toward same-sex relationships and do not expect to receive widespread support from the community at large. This need to remain in the closet or the fear of being humiliated keeps victims vulnerable to being targets and does not allow the perpetrator to receive punishment.

16. What does age have to do with sexual harassment?

Although anyone regardless of their age can experience sexual harassment, age can be a strong predictive factor. In fact, research suggests that age is one of the most important predictors of one's risk for sexual harassment (and sexual assault). Certain age groups can be identified to have a high frequency of sexual behavior, which puts them at risk for a whole host of issues. Sexually transmitted infections (STIs), unwanted sexual attention, and sexual assault would all be more likely with that increased focus on sexual activity.

Specifically, it is not surprising to recognize that our adolescent population are more vulnerable to sexual behaviors. Teenagers aged 13–18 are likely to face high school culture with constant exposure to sexual comments and potential for sexual harassment. Some high school students are the target of bullying that takes on a sexual nature.

College students can be another logical group who are at increased risk of sexual harassment. Whether students attending a university are living in dorms or in housing that is situated off campus, they are out of the home for the first time. This lack of supervision coupled with a focus on romantic relationships—dating and casual hookups—amps up the tendency for sexual behaviors to occur. Unfortunately, this opens the door for unwanted sexual attention and sexual harassment to take place as well. The data suggests that these students on college campuses are at increased risk for contracting sexually transmitted infections. College students are most commonly diagnosed with the following STIs: human papillomavirus (HPV), chlamydia, and HSV-2 genital herpes. Of the college students, the youngest (freshman year) were most likely to be diagnosed and treated for STIs. For example, the prevalence of chlamydia among students who were freshmen in college was above 13 percent compared to under 10 percent (9.7 percent) for students across all years of the university experience.

While high school and college students are logically "at-risk" groups, a surprising trend was seen in older adults who reported high levels of sexual activity. Health educators have speculated that this spike in sexual behavior among older adults was associated with the perception that contraception was not needed to prevent pregnancy. Older adults in retirement communities also reported having proximity and increased access to sexual partners. Some older adults adopted a fatalistic viewpoint of "I'm going to die anyway," which made them more likely to engage in unprotected sexual activity. Further, while the jury is still out and more research is needed to understand the rate of sexual harassment within this group, it stands to reason that increased sexual behavior is associated with an opportunity for unwanted sexual attention. It is likely that this generation might be least likely to report sexual harassment when it does take place due to generational influences on mindsets around the norms of acceptable behavior. Therefore, it will take time to obtain an accurate estimate for the older adult population.

While certain age groups might be more at risk for being the victims of sexual harassment, differences were also found with respect to attitudes about what was considered sexual harassment in the workplace. One study found that older employees had a higher likelihood of reporting the presence of pinups in the office or making jokes of a sexual nature as sexual harassment than their younger counterparts. On a related note, employees who had been at the job for a longer time were more likely to characterize sexual jokes as sexual harassment than those individuals with a shorter tenure. Both men and women who were older were more likely to hold supervisory positions. From an attitudinal perspective, a critical piece of information gleaned in a 2005 study was that older men were more likely to say that women do not really mean "no" when they say "no" than younger male employees.

Another notable difference in the workplace is related to one's knowledge of existing policies around sexual harassment. Specifically, older employees were found to have much more knowledge than their younger counterparts with respect to the organization's sexual harassment policies and procedures. Likewise, older employees reported at a higher rate than younger ones that they had experienced sexual harassment and as a result felt victimized.

One study that involved surveying almost 600 municipal employees broke down findings by age category and found that there were group differences by age across women. For example, in the 30–39 years and 30 and under category, women seemed to hold significantly different views from the 40–49 years old women and women over 50 years of age with respect to experiences and attitudes about sexual harassment.

Female employees who were younger than 30 years of age were unlikely to serve in supervisory or leadership positions at the time of the study. These younger employees did not seem to think that the sexual harassment training they had received was effective. Interestingly, a generational gap was exhibited for views about what constituted sexual harassment. The youngest women in the sample did not label many of the behaviors as severe enough to be characterized as sexual harassment. Furthermore, these young women did not express feeling victimized when they were the recipient of such behaviors. Women younger than 30 years of age were opposed to publicizing sexual harassment complaints and possible punishments. They were dissatisfied with how previous sexual harassment cases were handled in the workplace in so far as how the accused individuals were treated.

Women aged 30–39 years were less likely to report having experienced sexual harassment than the older age groups. They denied experiencing hostile work environment in their current positions and seemed to lack the personal knowledge about sexual harassment possessed by the women in the 40–49 age group and the over 50 age group. These women lacked formal training about the organization's policies and procedures on how to address sexual harassment. They (women 30–39 years) did not believe female employees were using their physical attractiveness to get ahead and gain promotions within the workplace.

Women over the age of 40 years were much more likely than the younger groups (under 30 years old, 30–39 years old) to report being victims of sexual harassment. This tendency to have more experience of sexual harassment might be attributed to holding a broader definition of what behaviors should count as sexual harassment. Women aged 40–49 years reported that current sexual harassment policies endorsed maintaining confidentiality of those individuals who had been accused of sexual harassment.

As previously stated, older age was associated with having a longer tenure at one's job. For women in the older than 50 years old category, they were more likely to have achieved a supervisory status and to have been on the job longer than younger employees. These women (over 50 years old category) reported sexual harassment at higher rates than the other groups of female employees. Although the women older than 50 years admitted to experiencing sexual harassment and hostile work environment in previous employment settings, they did not tend to report sexual harassment in their current position. A possible explanation for this age-related trend could be that women experience sexual harassment as they are climbing the career ladder. Once these women over 50 years of age become supervisors, they regain control of their destiny and can influence the workplace culture and environment (e.g., level of tolerance for certain behaviors, presence of pinups). This older group of female employees were satisfied about how sexual harassment complaints were being handled and felt punishments should be publicized in order to prevent future acts of sexual harassment. Women over 50 years of age also reported feeling confident about how to address cases when they came up and had received effective training in how to maintain confidentiality.

When considering the intersection of gender and age for male employees, some interesting findings emerged for these groups. Men younger than 30 years of age were much less likely to be supervisors than men in other age categories. The youngest men denied knowing of people or being exposed themselves to sexual harassment. They reported it was unlikely they would report behaviors if they occurred. The youngest men seemed unclear about what constitutes sexual harassment and lacked knowledge about organizational policies and procedures to address hostile work environment.

Men in the 30–39 years old age group were less likely to hold supervisory roles than male employees of 40–49 years of age or those 50 and older. Like the men under 30 years of age, men in this age category were unfamiliar with the policies and had received little training. They also lacked confidence about the definition of sexual harassment. To this end, men in this age group were more likely to have received compliments and invitations to go out on dates than men from other age categories. These behaviors were not viewed by men aged 30–39 years of age as sexual harassment, and therefore, they did not express feeling victimized when they were the recipients of such attention.

Men in the 40–49 age group tended to more likely experience being the victim of sexual harassment than men in other age categories. Moreover, they were more likely to have reported sexual harassment when it occurred. This tendency may be a product of their attitude that sexual harassment is a serious problem. These men also admitted to feeling like a victim rather than feeling flattered when they received unwanted attention in the workplace. This group of men supported having strong and decisive policies around sexual harassment as well as confidentiality for both the accused and accuser.

Men over 50 years of age reported feeling confident about the training they had received on how to manage sexual harassment complaints. As expected, these older men were more likely to serve in supervisory roles than their younger male counterparts. Additionally, these men were able to describe cases they had handled in a supervisory capacity. Like the women in this age bracket, men over 50 reported being knowledgeable about their organization's policies and procedures for dealing with sexual harassment. In summary, regardless of gender age was a predictor for holding a supervisory role in one's organization and was correlated with possessing more knowledge of policies and procedures around sexual harassment. This age group was also most likely to have received necessary training to identify the definition of sexual harassment (as a broad spectrum of sexual behaviors) and felt more confident addressing complaints when they emerged. On the flip side, age did appear to be a predictor of having firsthand experience of sexual harassment as a victim or a supervisor. Therefore, it can be underscored that both age and gender (as well as the intersection of the two) are strong influences and can impact risk for sexual harassment.

17. What do race or ethnicity have to do with sexual harassment?

Given the connection between sexual harassment and power, there is the potential for underrepresented groups of social categories such as class, race, and gender to be at increased risk for victimization. Gender and age have been covered in previous questions; however, there are some parallels between the phenomenon of gender discrimination as a microcosm of power in society (and how sexual harassment is used as a weapon against girls and women) and what happens with respect to race and ethnicity. Furthermore, it is important to note that the intersections of gender and race must be examined when considering one's potential risk for sexual harassment.

The term "white privilege" has been used to characterize the subtle and obvious ways that life experiences may be different for people based on the color of one's skin. Stereotypes associated with the color of one's skin can contribute to inequalities related to opportunities for advancement in one's organization, increased likelihood of being harassed, and higher risk for financial difficulties. Having the potential of racial or ethnic discrimination for being a person of color sets one up for a variety of abuses across the setting whether it be school, one's workplace, or out in public.

An early attempt in 1981 to study one's race and risk for sexual harassment did not reveal significant differences among White, Hispanic, and African American women. By contrast, men who were in minority groups such as African American and Native American reported higher rates of sexual harassment. As studies have continued in this area, results are not conclusive. Some research indicates that African American women respond similarly (around 44 percent) to their white female counterparts or even report fewer instances of unwanted requests of a sexual nature. One study found that 34 percent of African American women reported experiencing sexual harassment at least once, whereas 53 percent of white women reported at least one incident. Researchers have hypothesized that this difference may have reflected a trend for underreporting among African American women, associated with lack of power and belief that action would be taken after filing a complaint.

A Department of Defense-funded study indicated that one at-risk group that emerged was of Native American participants—both men and women, who seemed to report higher rates of sexual harassment than the other racial groups. Specifically, 50 percent of Native American participants reported experiencing sexual harassment behaviors compared with African American, Hispanic, white, and Asian American participants who comprised around 36 percent. Ultimately, when taking gender into account Native American women were most susceptible to sexual harassing behaviors with African American and Hispanic women next most likely to experience sexual harassment. Asian American and white targets seemed to experience less harassment.

Researchers have since underscored the higher rates of sexual harassment for African American individuals, which are predictive of these power dynamics in society. It was also noted that African American victims were more likely be blamed as responsible for the attack (e.g., sexual assault, rape) and/or being the target of sexually harassing behaviors. It was also found that African American women were stereotyped as being promiscuous. These societal biases led to charges being taken less seriously when African American women experienced sexual harassment.

For example, one statistic showed that African American girls had a higher likelihood of experiencing sexual harassment than Caucasian girls of the same age. While both were often the targets of sexual harassment, 49 percent of African American girls (compared to 37 percent of Caucasian girls) reported that their clothes had been pulled on by perpetrators.

Other forms of harassment demonstrated similar trends: 48 percent African American versus 36 percent Caucasian girls reported being cornered and 30 percent African American versus 22 percent Caucasian females were forced to kiss someone.

When African American girls graduated from high school, sexual harassment would not cease to exist. In fact, African American women were disproportionately likely to file sexual harassment complaints in the workplace. Related to the workplace setting, one study found that African American employees were much more likely to report that receiving pressure for unwanted sexual activity was characterized as sexual harassment than individuals who self-identified in a different race or ethnic category.

18. Does being a victim of childhood abuse increase one's likelihood of experiencing sexual harassment as an adult?

There is evidence that being a victim of childhood trauma is a risk factor for a variety of mental health conditions. For example, adults who were exposed to sexual abuse as children are found to be vulnerable for developing disordered eating and eating disorders later in life. There are a few explanations for this correlation, but the relationship is complicated and not easy to define.

First, early experiences of childhood trauma will inevitably have a negative impact on a person's self-worth and how they internalize their values and feelings of inadequacy. A pattern of blaming oneself for being abused is common. Feelings of guilt and shame are frequently reported by adults who acknowledge they were victims of incest, rape, or sexual trauma. As a child, there is no circumstance in which experiencing sexual abuse or any other type of childhood abuse (verbal or physical) is appropriate or anything except wrong, but the child has a warped sense of self. There is some evidence that children who are approached by adult perpetrators are selected for being "people pleasers" or being compliant. Realistically, no child is immune to being abused since perpetrators seek out an opportunity to infiltrate the lives of their victims. An adult who has experienced abuse in their past may tolerate or accept unwanted sexual advances to a greater degree than someone who has not had this childhood trauma, if they view it as normal.

It is important to note that for children who do report that they have been abused, the response to their report is critical for their response later in life to subsequent events. For example, if the child reporting sexual abuse was not believed by an adult or no action was taken against the perpetrator, that incident will have an intensely negative impact later in life. That same child will almost certainly be less likely to report the next time abuse happens (or as an adult when sexual harassment takes place). By contrast, if a child reports a negative event has occurred and is told by an adult emphatically that that behavior was inappropriate and action is taken, the child might be less likely to blame themselves for the abuse (and thus internalize their role in the event). In summary, children learn early on how to cope with traumatic events and if or when it is safe to speak up. Therefore, ensuring that children have resources and a safe place to turn to is essential for helping victims early in life.

19. What is victim blaming?

One of the biggest problems with addressing sexual harassment is the tendency for incidents to go unreported. In some cases, the victim will wait until much later to report and the perpetrator goes unpunished. Experiences that occur are deeply personal and create internal conflict. Victims also blame themselves, ironically enough, for somehow inviting the behavior. Despite the turmoil experienced when one is victimized, they know deep down that they were wronged, and sadly, the pattern of sexual harassment continues with the same or different victims. Once a victim decides to come forward, they will face a whole other layer of scrutiny from others when they file a complaint. The victim will likely face being on trial for one's character and risk being in the media spotlight. In worse-case scenario, some victims have even faced death threats, been demoted, or lost their jobs.

Victim blaming is defined as holding the victim partially or completely responsible for the wrongful act (such as sexual harassment) committed against them. Blaming the victim frequently occurs in sexual harassment when there is a perceived benefit (e.g., job promotion) for the victim. However, girls and women are often accused of "asking for it" (i.e., sexual harassment) by dressing in a particular way or behaving in a certain manner. In other words, sexual harassment is attributed to the victim rather than the perpetrator. In the 2019 film *Bombshell*, a young woman dressed in a tight black dress in Fox News goes to a meeting with CEO Roger Ailes. She is asked to "twirl" and raise her dress in a clear instance of sexual harassment. Because sexual harassment often occurs when only the victim and the perpetrator are present, it can be hard to prove. Literally, when a report is made it becomes a "he said, she said" scenario. The victim may be blamed for being overly flirtatious or too friendly. Or they may be accused of drinking too much.

These age-old explanations for sexual harassment let the perpetrators off the hook and serve to normalize the inappropriate behaviors at school or one's workplace. In fact, many perpetrators have attorneys who success-fully dismiss the sexual harassment claims if they can show that they are engaging in a consensual relationship with the victim. Unfortunately, vic-tim blaming makes the report of sexual harassment less likely and creates a culture that is hostile and uncomfortable for the person forced to suffer in silence. For someone in high school who has faced sexual harassment, they may have to change schools to escape the abusive behavior.

It is not uncommon in workplace sexual harassment for the person to leave their job even if it jeopardizes their career. Ultimately, the sad reality is that the victim will not escape unscathed from reporting their experiences. Victims often feel faced with a bind, letting their perpetra-tor go on without receiving consequences for their actions. But if one reports the incident, they face a firestorm of uncertainty. Therefore, vic-tims are advised to proceed with caution, plenty of support, and ample documentation.

20. What is sex addiction? Is there a relationship between sex addiction and sexual harassment?

Sex addiction refers to a disordered way of viewing intimacy that is pro-gressive and dangerous. A person experiences compulsive thoughts and behaviors around sexual acts that are highly negative. These may involve obtaining and viewing pornographic material, indulging in legal and ille-gal behaviors, and being highly destructive. Although sex addiction is often misunderstood as a "love for sex" or "can't get enough," it is a serious mental health condition like other forms of addiction. If not treated, the condition will get progressively worse and more severe, and the sex addict will go to unimaginable lengths to get their "fix." It is important to note that sex addiction is completely distinct from sexual harassment.

Sexual harassment has erroneously been mistaken for a way for per-petrators to act out sexual urges or a form of sexual attraction. The issue is confounded with the tendency for victims to be blamed for being the target of unwanted sexual attention due to wearing revealing clothing or engaging in flirtatious banter. In fact, the negative behavior rarely, if ever, has anything to do with sex. Sexual addiction is defined as having a compulsion to engage in sexual acts that leads to risky behavior such as extramarital sexual activity, sex with prostitutes, and anonymous sex.

As with other kinds of addictions (e.g., substance use, alcohol, gambling, exercise), sex addicts develop an increasing tolerance for and escalating urge to engage in their compulsions related to sexual activity. Therefore, sex addicts are obsessive and seek out opportunities to engage in their compulsion even when it jeopardizes their monogamous relationship or puts them at risk for developing a sexually transmitted infection. They feel compelled to act on their urges and are unable to release the pressure until they have engaged in the compulsion. However, the feeling of relief is short lived, and to break the cycle, sex addicts must seek treatment.

Studies have demonstrated that sexual harassment is about gaining or exerting power or influence over another person. For sexual harassment at one's school, it may be about bullying another classmate of the same or different gender. If a power dynamic exists like a teacher-student relationship, sexual harassment involves abusing one's authority and violating the standards of appropriate ways to interact with students by making advances or comments. However, the teacher does not necessarily have sex addiction simply because they act in a sexual manner toward a student. In most cases, this power differential is about control and has little to do with sexual attraction or compulsion of certain acts.

Consequences and Effects

21. What are the physical effects associated with sexual harassment?

Symptoms and warning signs of sexual harassment are related to the overall consequences of being a victim of sexual harassment. In other words, many of those "red flags" can represent short- and long-term effects of sexual harassment. It is noteworthy that the consequences of sexual harassment span from experiencing physical effects to making an impact on one's academic record or performance as an employee. Sexual harassment, like other forms of traumatic life experiences, is not easily forgotten, and the consequences emerge in many ways.

Impacts on one's physical health may be short term or may impose longer lasting effects on the body. From a health promotion standpoint, sexual harassment is harmful to the functioning of bodily systems. For example, individuals with a history of sexual harassment and assault were found to have greater risk of high blood pressure and high triglycerides and to suffer from poor sleep quality than those individuals who do not experience sexual harassment. Sleep disturbances were a common effect of sexual harassment during the experience and beyond that. Victims of sexual harassment may frequently report difficulties in falling or staying asleep (i.e., insomnia) as well as the presence of nightmares. Unfortunately, an inadequate amount of sleep or poor sleep quality is tied to a host of other health problems.

One such health problem, heart health, has also been associated with sexual harassment. Specifically, researchers from the University of Pittsburgh investigated the relationship between heart disease and trauma. These researchers discovered that women who experienced traumatic events during their life such as sexual harassment exhibited heart and blood vessel functioning that was poorer than individuals who did not report having traumatic experiences. This impaired functioning could put these victims of sexual harassment at increased risk for significant health problems, such as cardiovascular issues. Another explanation for the heightened risk for heart health issues was the presence of stress hormones triggered by sexual harassment. Sexual harassment is perceived as a threat by one's brain, which can cause one's stress hormones (i.e., cortisol) to rise sharply. This less-than-conscious fight-or-flight response causes a person to feel anxious or off-kilter. When cortisol levels remain at a high level (associated with being in a constant state of stress), one's physical health is intensely impacted. These chronically elevated cortisol levels can cause inflammation to happen in the body. Unfortunately, inflammation has been tied to many disease states such as cancers and cardiovascular disease. Stress has also been tied to acute physical symptoms such as stomach aches and ulcers and headaches including migraines. These physical effects can be misread, and victims of sexual harassment may not realize the connection of their symptoms to the stress in their lives.

Individuals could also be more susceptible to developing sexually transmitted diseases (STIs) such as genital warts and chlamydia. Interestingly, the presence of STIs or other genital infections among victims especially children and teenagers proved to be an effective way for some sexual harassment cases to be detected. Some children may develop bedwetting behaviors or may soil the bed. It is also possible to observe bruising on the body or unexplained bleeding with sexual assault.

Another physical effect of sexual harassment is related to changes in body weight or size. A victim may display marked weight gain—likely associated with binge eating episodes and emotional eating—that involves significant pounds in a relatively short period of time. Excessive eating will likely entail highly accessible binge foods that are high in salt or sugar content. Likewise, another potential effect of sexual harassment is weight loss. A person who suffers from sexual harassment may restrict food, lose appetite, or develop patterns of disordered eating. Individuals with a history of trauma are more likely to show signs of clinical eating disorders.

22. What are the psychological/emotional effects associated with sexual harassment? What role does sexual harassment play in the development of eating disorders or other mental health disorders?

Although the physical effects are well documented and significant, there are equally severe consequences of sexual harassment on one's psychological and emotional health. In fact, the mental aspects in sexual harassment are likely the most enduring and lasting for the victim. A recent case of an incident involving Dr. Christine Blasey Ford and Supreme Court nominee Brett Kavanaugh allegedly happened over 30 years ago; however, the psychological damage still lingered. Dr. Ford described experiencing anxiety and post-traumatic stress disorder, which are both commonly cited among victims of sexual harassment. Unfortunately, the triggers associated with one's anxiety disorder or post-traumatic stress disorder may lead victims to develop certain phobias or extreme avoidance. One finding was that victims of sexual harassment were less likely to visit the doctor or dentist than individuals who had not experienced a history of sexual trauma. Moreover, findings in the *Journal of American Medical Association* indicated that women with a history had double risk of developing anxiety disorders.

Mood changes are both a warning sign and effect of sexual harassment. For individuals experiencing sexual harassment, they face increased likelihood of having depression and may likely become withdrawn from daily activities such as family, school, and work obligations.

It was estimated that individuals with a history of sexual trauma were three times as likely to develop a depressive disorder. A study that focused on sexual harassment in the workplace found that individuals who were sexually harassed by colleagues in the workplace (e.g., supervisors, subordinates, or peers) exhibited more severe depression symptoms than individuals who experienced harassment from customers or clients. While neither form of harassment is a good thing, it is likely that those harassed by their colleagues feel powerless and have a harder time coping. A client or customer may seem like a necessary part of dealing with the job or something more temporary. The tendency to avoid school or work was associated with job losses or not achieving one's potential. This negative effect on one's ability to function carried on even when the individual was no longer in the setting in which sexual harassment took place. Some initial research on men and women in the military found that individuals who reported sexual trauma were more at risk of being homeless following their deployment due to an inability to form relationships, to function, and to hold down a job.

Some of the emotional effects that are not readily identified by the victim but are meaningful include self-doubt, blaming oneself, humiliation, anger, and loss of trust. Self-doubt can emerge initially when a victim of sexual harassment experiences confusion over what has happened. There might be a tendency to try to find a reason for the bad behavior of one's boss, coworker, or peer in school—"What did I do to deserve this?" This response is tied to a disbelief that someone would willingly treat someone else so poorly and to rationalize the situation. There may also be a strong feeling that one must persist despite the adversity or poor treatment one is receiving. Being raised to overcome challenges and "stay the course" may result in an employee staying in a hostile work environment.

Victims often tend to blame themselves for sexual harassment. They may feel powerless and show denial about what has happened. There is also a tendency to feel they did not exert a sense of control or confront their perpetrator sooner to stop the sexual harassment. Instead of taking legal action, many victims will try to change their behavior. For example, some women will dress more conservatively, wear glasses, or gain weight to appear undesirable to the opposite sex or one's perpetrator. For victims of trauma, the extra weight can add as protection or safety from the abuse.

Humiliation is another common emotional response to sexual harassment. Unfortunately, sexual harassment often results in the victim feeling devalued and demeaned. This feeling of humiliation contributes to a decreased motivation at work due to receiving attention of a sexual nature rather than for one's job performance. Due to the intense embarrassment associated with the negative behaviors, it is common for self-esteem to plunge, and victims also hesitate to come forward to report sexual harassment.

Another emotional reaction that is difficult to deal with for those who have a history of sexual harassment is anger. While anger may be a tough emotion to express in a healthy way within one's families, when it comes to sexual harassment, angry outbursts may occur unexpectedly. This anger can fester and lead to the desire to get revenge or be violent against one's harasser. Victims of sexual harassment have admitted to wanting to burn the house down of their perpetrator or to make the person suffer by telling their family members. Anger is often tricky because it is uncovered suddenly after memories have been repressed for months or even years. With the #MeToo movement, many individuals uncovered the realization that they too had been a victim of sexual harassment.

While knowledge is power, those victims also must cope with intense emotions such as anger. Being able to express anger and channel this emotion in a healthy way can be accomplished with counseling and working through issue of sexual harassment. It is important not to continue to "stuff feelings back down" or they will come out unexpectedly and likely negative ways.

Loss of trust is an emotional effect of sexual harassment that spills over into other relationships with the same and opposite sex. Because trust has been violated in sexual harassment, there may be a tendency to displace negative emotions to one's significant other or spouse. A person who experiences sexual harassment may also refuse to trust dates moving forward. This lack of trust can inevitably impact the quality of one's sexual relationships that rely heavily on trust and commitment.

It is common for eating patterns to change among individuals who suffer from sexual harassment. Eating is highly psychological in nature and often tied to one's mood. Therefore, it is unsurprising perhaps that when one is feeling depressed or disempowered, they will eat less or more than what is normal. While a short-term change might be expected and even viewed as a maladaptive coping strategy, having a history of trauma has also been predictive of developing more severe mental health disorders. Individuals who have been clinically diagnosed with eating disorders (anorexia nervosa, bulimia nervosa, binge eating disorder) have a higher likelihood of having a history of trauma than individuals without an eating disorder. Furthermore, individuals who experience sexual harassment have also been found to report lower self-esteem and poorer body image as a direct effect.

In extreme cases, the person affected by sexual harassment may exhibit self-harming or suicidal tendencies associated with the negative mental health effects. They may feel it is too difficult to keep living or self-worth may be compromised immensely. Therefore, it is important that individuals who have experienced sexual harassment be assessed for mood changes, depression, and clinical disorders and monitored for suicide risk.

23. How are academics impacted by sexual harassment?

Sexual harassment can have far-reaching effects when it comes to physical and psychological health, but there are also impacts on one's performance in the school or work setting. As would be expected of someone experiencing a high stress situation, one's ability to perform to their best ability will likely be impaired. For victims of sexual harassment, one's concentration is often negatively impacted as they are distracted with worries about receiving unwanted comments and behaviors in school.

There are many consequences related to academics associated with sexual harassment. If a person is experiencing sexual harassment at school, they may want to avoid the experience or risk of sexual harassment entirely. This may mean that the victim skips classes or does not want to attend school for fear of additional exposure. In fact, a student who previously had perfect attendance may stay home or cut class just to protect themselves from harm associated with sexual harassment. When a student has a choice to eliminate certain classes from their schedule, they may opt to drop the class (e.g., physical education) in which sexual harassment is occurring.

It is not surprising that the distraction from sexual harassment often impacts one's grades. Some students reported having difficulty concentrating during class lectures, whereas other students scored lower test grades. Further, one's confidence in their educational ability and motivation to study decreased as a consequence of sexual harassment. In some cases, victims of sexual harassment reported that their confidence suffered so much that they felt they lacked the ability to graduate from high school or to continue on to a university. This impact is not trivial as one's entire career trajectory could be altered by suffering grades and a negative academic record.

Some students were so negatively affected by the sexual harassment that they pushed to change schools. The ability to change schools is influenced by a myriad of factors including economic and geographical issues, but some students did successfully switch schools. The impact on the family as a result of this school change was the need for transportation (if school was at a farther distance) or costs associated with private schooling. In extreme cases, families were forced to relocate to enable their son or daughter to move to a different school within the district.

Teachers and school administrators have grappled with how to better address and prevent bullying in the schools. There is broad awareness that such behaviors (which include sexual harassment) have harmful effects including increased risk for suicide. For teachers who are already concerned about growing class sizes, the presence of sexual harassment and bullying creates yet another barrier to the ideal learning environment. When a situation necessitates school intervention by teacher or administrator, their attention is divided such that not only is the victim affected by also the rest of the students.

24. How is one's job performance and satisfaction impacted by sexual harassment?

In addition to having personal consequences of both a psychological and physical nature, it is important to consider the impact of sexual harassment on one's job. Individuals who are falling victim to sexual harassment will not want to be continually subjected to negative treatment at one's place of employment. It is likely that they will suffer loss of morale and motivation, which would negatively impact one's job satisfaction. Further, there are innumerable consequences around one's job status and performance.

For a person experiencing a hostile work environment, they will undoubtedly face a myriad of negative emotions. While depression and anxiety are common for an employee who is experiencing sexual harassment, it is also likely that they will be more distracted and less focused on the task at hand. This decrease in focus and lack of concentration can result in making more mistakes on the job, performing tasks with lower accuracy, or decreasing one's efficiency at completing the task. In addition, the worker may be more likely to miss days and accrue excessive absences. This tendency to miss work can negatively impact benefits by draining sick days and vacation pay, or depending on the position, it might be associated with lower pay (if an hourly employee). An employee who is experiencing sexual harassment may avoid certain meetings, social outings, or projects that are crucial for one's advancement or success on the job. Unfortunately, those tremendous effects on one's job performance can impact their performance reviews negatively and create risk of disciplinary notice or losing one's job.

Alarmingly, it is also possible that an employee who does not accept the advances of one's supervisor may face negative retaliation of a subtle or more direct nature. Perhaps the employee may no longer be invited to certain meetings or assigned to projects with high value to the company. In more severe instances, that employee might be demoted or even fired (with one's employer offering performance reasons). That is why it is so important to report sexual harassment when it has occurred rather than in response to actions by one's employer.

Sometimes an employee may be reassigned to another department or unit to prevent further sexual harassment from taking place. This change or reassignment is not always viewed positively by the employee (despite being out of the crosshairs of sexual harassment). When an employee suffers from sexual harassment over a period of weeks, months, or even years, the outcome is almost always negative. Ultimately, they may leave or quit before having another job in place or may accept a job at lower pay to escape the negative work environment.

25. What are the economic effects associated with sexual harassment?

It is important to note that in addition to consequences suffered at the individual level for victims of sexual harassment, there are economic implications. Someone may face the reality of needing to leave a job prematurely due to experiencing a hostile work environment, unwanted attention of a sexual nature, or fear of retaliation. Certainly, if a person does this without having another job lined up or is in a position of feeling the need to accept a lower-paying job, there is the strong potential for economic loss. Individuals may also experience economic consequences associated with health care bills related to stress and illness tied to sexual harassment.

At an organizational level, employers also experience costs related to sexual harassment. In fact, an earlier report provided by the Merit Systems Protection Board suggested that the federal government lost $189 million due to sexual harassment over a two-year timeframe ending in 1980. According to the 1994 United States Merit Systems Protection Board study, the cost to the federal government jumped to $325 million due to sexual harassment. Why were there losses? These dollar amounts represent both a drop in work productivity and the tendency for a higher turnover to occur in the presence of sexual harassment. These outcomes, estimated to be $36.7 million, resulted in the need to hire and train new employees (because of replacing employees who had left their jobs due to sexual harassment). Moreover, when employees left their jobs there was the additional cost for employers as they had to pay out sick leave for missed time on the job (estimated to be $26.1 million) as well as reduced productivity at the individual and group levels (approximately $204.5 million). A study conducted in the late 1980s demonstrated that each of the Fortune 500 companies experienced a total annual cost of nearly $7 million due to sexual harassment. These numbers well exceeded the cost of implementing a sexual harassment prevention program. Furthermore, even though it is sometimes difficult to quantify, many employers report that sexual harassment hurts business, image, and brand loyalty.

In a more recent article published in 2017 by the *Harvard Business Review*, clearly the economic impact of sexual harassment remains a reality in many places of employment. Women in a variety of industries from politics to technology may leave their jobs, their companies, or their occupations if they experience sexual harassment. This tendency to exit one's industry or chosen career can severely undermine a person's earning power. Another unintended economic consequence may be related to the difficulty of landing another job at the same salary level. Leaving a job, especially if working for a small company, can hurt one's reputation and ability to score solid professional references.

In sum, the economic costs of sexual harassment span from direct costs to business due to loss of reputation or having to pay a settlement to an employee to more indirect types of cost. Indirect costs include the issue of absenteeism, loss of work productivity, and tendency for turnover in job positions.

26. What does it mean to be a "survivor" of sexual harassment?

Many individuals would rather be referred to as "survivors" than victims of sexual harassment. The word "victim" often conjures up some form of pity or, worse yet, might be associated with blame. What was the victim wearing, drinking, and doing out at that hour of the night? What was the victim's sexual history? In contrast, "survivor" denotes taking charge of one's destiny and being an advocate for others who have suffered similar forms of harassment. There is a suggestion of healing that might be implied if one is a survivor.

Yet, there is some debate over whether individuals who have experienced sexual harassment should even be called survivors. One provocative 2018 article entitled, "I'm not a sexual assault 'survivor'—I'm a victim," in *Harper's Bazaar* is written by an author who clearly eschews the term "survivor." She states in no uncertain terms that the label "survivor" seems to suggest a superhero or someone who was able to successfully overcome the monumental hurdle and challenge of experiencing sexual harassment. In the author's case, this term did not fit her daily experiences of someone who still suffers from the lasting effects of trauma (especially the emotional ones). A similar argument has been launched in the eating disorder and addiction communities regarding whether to call someone "in recovery" or "recovered." While for substance use disorders people are typically thought to always be in recovery, people who undergo eating disorder treatment may eventually achieve the past tense of recovery. For an individual to be considered "recovered," they must no longer engage in disordered eating behaviors and must develop a more positive body image. When triggers are experienced, a person who is recovered has healthy coping skills to address emotions as they arise. A similar mindset could be applied to a survivor of sexual harassment.

Ultimately, whether the label "survivor" is used, it should be underscored how difficult it can be to disclose that an event has happened. Being a survivor is often defined as owning that an experience has happened to them and taking the necessary steps to grow and move on. Taking action to stop the harassment when it is taking place is a necessary and important step for the healing process of a survivor. For a survivor, the memory will always be there of the sexual harassment, but the intense rage and strong emotions are somewhat muted. It is possible for the survivor to find a healthy workplace (or setting) free of sexual harassment and to speak up when something is not right. Ideally, being a survivor is like having "recovered" from a drug addiction, in that being a victim of sexual harassment is no longer a defining characteristic or primary part of one's identity.

Many survivors can benefit from the help of a mental health professional to discuss one's experiences and coping strategies to deal with triggers as they come up. Triggers refer to situations that can happen unexpectedly and can result in intense emotions associated with the memory of one's trauma or sexual harassment experience. A survivor may be surprised at the various emotions one experiences ranging from fear to anger toward one's perpetrator (or those who did not help) or intense sadness about the loss of a childhood, college experience, or job. A therapist can help survivors who are working through phobias and anxiety and developing interpersonal skills and strategies to be reintegrated as a healthy member of society.

If needed, one can be prescribed psychotropic medications for addressing depression, anxiety, or other clinical disorders. Survivors may find support in meeting others who have experienced sexual harassment in the form of support groups or organizations like RAINN (Rape, Abuse & Incest National Network) that provide a myriad of resources. RAINN offers information on the website as well as other resources that can be perused to learn more about what a person might expect if they have faced sexual harassment.

RAINN also offers resources for those who offer support to survivors of sexual harassment. The key points are to avoid judgement. Survivors will experience plenty of guilt and a tendency to blame oneself. As a support person for a survivor, it is important to know about the available resources and have the numbers of the National Sexual Assault Hotline or local support groups.

27. How does sexual harassment impact the perpetrator?

Earlier in this book, the common characteristics of a perpetrator were discussed. It was mentioned that profiles have been identified, but that in reality, anyone regardless of their social category (e.g., gender, race, ethnicity, size, socioeconomic status) or status within an organization (e.g., student, supervisor, or employee) can commit sexual harassment. This makes it difficult to openly categorize "who" is offending, and it means that actions are taken once the act has occurred rather than use a proactive approach to sexual harassment prevention.

However, one trend that has emerged from the literature suggests that many perpetrators have been victims themselves. The abuse cycle plays out, and in some cases, sexual harassment can be a learned behavior. For example, a person may observe a parent who treats the opposite sex poorly and makes gendered comments. This socialization regarding gender roles and how to treat other human beings may be internalized and may impact future action. In other words, the discriminatory behavior is normalized and seen as acceptable. Thus, the violation may be internalized as an outgrowth of this attitude toward treatment of others and acceptance of sexual harassment behaviors. This tendency for perpetrators to be victims can be a hard pill to swallow. Why would someone who suffered from abuse, trauma, and poor treatment possibly choose to inflict such negative behavior on someone else? Examples of victims (or survivors depending on which label one uses) are rampant among people who have experienced abuse and who turn around and abuse others due to poor coping resources. Perceptions of reality may be altered, and confusion around which behaviors are acceptable can play out in future interactions.

Feelings of entitlement have been observed with certain perpetrators. "I deserve this" or "you should want the attention" represent distorted beliefs that if acted on translate into sexual harassment. This can be uncomfortable when one's belief that "you should like this compliment about your body" is met with a negative response. Some perpetrators have used this distorted belief to attempt to blame the victim ("she was asking for the attention by wearing a dress that short") and to settle one's mental frame about the situation. A similar dissonance occurs when a perpetrator argues (and perhaps believes on some level) that sexual assault or harassment were somehow consensual.

Not much attention has been placed on the effects of sexual harassment on the perpetrator for obvious reasons. But the answer is highly dependent on the outcome and consequences of harassing. As seen in the high-profile cases of Weinstein and Bill Cosby, even rich and famous people can lose their jobs and be charged with offenses against the law. Being in a powerful, supervisory position and exerting one's authority over another employee is taken seriously in today's workplace. Many human resource departments are focused on training current and new employees about Title IX to prevent sexual harassment. Employees have been given more clear information about how to report instances when they happen.

Like the victim or survivor, the perpetrator will also face negative effects of sexual harassment. First, the perpetrator will risk facing employment consequences associated with being charged for sexual harassment. The accused may lose their job, be demoted, or transferred to another department. This charge will represent a negative mark on the employee's record moving forward. Whether found to be guilty or not, there will be a lingering bias toward the accused employee.

Being charged with sexual harassment might lead to additional accusations as we have seen happen with some very public cases such as that of Matt Lauer from *NBC Today Show*. Suddenly the charges seem to fall like dominos, and it can be increasingly difficult to stop the momentum. There may be financial costs associated with job loss, legal costs, or paying out victims. There will be the potential for criminal investigation and to receive additional penalties (e.g., fines or prison time).

In addition to economic impacts, there may be social effects on the violator's relationship with their family. When sexual harassments become publicized, the family can be thrust into the media spotlight. People may judge the significant other or watch the reaction of family members. If found or suspected to be guilty, the accused perpetrator's infidelity may be uncovered. There may be relationship hardships and the potential for separation, divorce, or at the minimum turmoil and fighting within the current relationship. If the perpetrator has children, it will be difficult for them to process and handle the negative attention they receive. A perpetrator may worry about the safety of their family members especially if the case becomes public in nature.

Someone charged with a crime may experience social isolation. They may find themselves being treated differently. Perhaps the perpetrator will no longer be invited to social occasions, informal office parties, or lunch dates. It may be difficult to go out in public to run one's typical errands if the case has received a lot of local or national attention. Over time, an accused perpetrator may suffer from psychological and physical health consequences.

Emotional effects from the stress on the perpetrator are similar to victims. No matter the source of stress, stress has a negative impact on one's physical and psychological health. Stress has been directly linked to disease conditions such as diabetes, cardiovascular illness, and cancers. It is likely that the perpetrator will experience sleep and eating disturbances. Perpetrators are also likely to be vulnerable to the development of anxiety, depression, and other mood disorders. They may face increased risk of self-harming behaviors (e.g., cutting) or suicide. Finally, this person will need to grapple with issues surrounding one's identity. This concept of "who am I" can change when one has been charged with a crime even if they are not found guilty. Will this criminalization be internalized and impact one's self-esteem? Whether one embraces the label as "perpetrator" or not, this will affect the person's attitude, behavior, and actions moving forward.

Confronting and Preventing Sexual Harassment

28. How is sexual harassment detected or reported?

While each school has a slightly different process when sexual harassment has taken place, the same basic procedure is typically followed within K-12 schools and university campuses. A sexual harassment incident is detected when a report is filed at the school. A Title IX coordinator or a school employee who is assigned to handle Title IX investigations will receive the complaint of sexual harassment. Once the complaint has been made, the Title IX coordinator will conduct an initial interview with the victim and/or the witness (if that is the person who was a bystander during the incident). The person who filed the complaint will be asked to provide details of what happened with as much specificity as possible. The Title IX coordinator of the school provides information regarding the process itself and victim rights. In addition, there may be a need to provide provisional steps to help the victim feel safe in the meantime. Moreover, the victim will be offered referrals for counseling and support services available within this initial interview session. Usually, following the initial interview with the school official, an investigator is assigned to the case. The identified perpetrator who is believed to have harmed or harassed will be contacted by the investigator to get their side of the story.

It is possible that the investigator may also follow up with the victim as well as any additional witnesses who come to light regarding the sexual harassment incident.

At the college level, after the investigation interviews are completed summaries will be sent to the witness and the accused perpetrator for their review. During the evidence review, either party can speak up to make corrections and clarifications or can oppose statements that are perceived to be false as stated by the other party or witnesses. This step can also provide the opportunity to comment on any evidence and its relevance to the case.

The next step for handling a complaint of sexual harassment involves issuing a determination about the validity of the complaint. When the evidence review has been completed, the investigator then confers a decision about whether the violation took place. In order to make the determination, the investigator must weigh what is referred to as a "preponderance of the evidence." This statement means that there should be sufficient evidence that sexual harassment likely took place. If the investigator reaches this conclusion and the school concurs that sexual harassment happened, a sanction may be recommended that represents a consequence for the person accused of harming the victim. At the college level, depending on the state and a variety of factors (such as whether the other party is a student or staff member), there may be a hearing once the determination is reached. Depending on the circumstances, the victim may or may not have the right to be present at the hearing. The other party may ask questions during this hearing about the alleged incident.

Another important piece to consider is that at the college level there is often an option to appeal once a conclusion has been reached about the sexual harassment claim as well as the proposed disciplinary action. For this option to appeal, one or both parties may contact the chancellor (president of the college/university) or another designated official of the university. Appeals are likely when the disciplinary action is viewed as inappropriate for the case—too large or too small. Another scenario that may influence an appeal is when the evidence is not seen to substantiate the finding or if there was a procedural error in the investigator or hearing. Finally, if there is new evidence that has come to light that should be considered for the decision, an appeal might be warranted. Once the appeal takes place, the case might be returned to the original investigator assigned to the case for review as well as to fix any errors made. Ultimately, the decision may be overturned (and replaced with new determination) or might be retained.

For cases that involve sexual harassment in K-12, the option to appeal and the specific procedure varies by state. The school district may have a unique appeal process if the outcome of the investigation is undesirable. In some cases, an appeal is made to a state entity such as the Department of Education within the person's state.

29. What are statutes of limitations?

It is common when talking about legal issues to hear the term "statutes of limitations." The statutes of limitations refer to the allowable time frame in which a person can file a complaint after an event has occurred that is allowable for legal recourse and action. In other words, how long can a person wait before they bring charges or a lawsuit against someone for something that has happened to them? In general, this could be any type of lawsuit, but for sexual harassment, having a designated timeframe is impactful for the victim and the potential success of the case. This restriction on when someone must file is compounded by the fact that many victims remain in denial, may experience shame, blame themselves, or be afraid to report due to anticipated retaliation.

Further complications are associated with the setting in which harassment has occurred and the fact that repressed memories may reappear for victims of sexual harassment. Unfortunately, for many individuals who have experienced sexual harassment it is not until they leave their place of employment or school that they feel safe to make a complaint against their harasser.

Civil law systems dictate that this prescriptive period represents the maximum time that can take place beyond the sexual harassment. The specified time frame (that is the maximum length of time since the sexual harassment) can vary from state to state. There are also some nuances related to when the crime happened (such as if the victim was a minor at the time). There are differences in civil action versus a criminal lawsuit as well.

For example, in the state of California there are multiple timelines for filing cases that involve sexual assault or harassment. In looking at taking civil action to recover damages associated with sexual harassment, an adult plaintiff faces a different time frame. Adults must file within 10 years from the date of the last reported incident of sexual harassment involving the defendant or within 3 years from the date that an injury or illness was discovered. This new statute of limitations for adults in California was revised to protect the victims and became official on January 1, 2019. For children in California, a new, broader set of statutes of limitations came into effect as of January 2020. Specifically, victims who are children can file civil lawsuits up until they turn 40 years of age. The range for discovery was increased from 3 years to 5 years for children.

If a person is making a claim against a school district or other government entity in California, there are different time limits. The filing is referred to as a "government claim" and might be as brief as six months for the maximum time limit from the occurrence of the incident whether you are a child or adult. Because of discrepancies in cases and states, it is important to check with the specific regulations for your state and seek legal counsel to navigate the process. It is important not to delay in filing as the rules are strict and waiting longer can sometimes have a negative effect on the outcome of one's case.

30. What steps should I take if I'm being sexually harassed?

First, you must acknowledge that it is not your fault above all else. When someone is sexually harassed, it is common to feel a variety of intense emotions including shame, anger, and embarrassment. Many victims tend to shoulder the blame or question themselves by wondering whether they did something to provoke the inappropriate behavior. Feelings of hopelessness or the desire to run away, change schools, or quit one's job is natural. It is important for someone who experiences sexual harassment, however, to take back the power. Most sexual harassment cases are not reported, so there are specific steps one should consider when they have been wronged in this way. Remember that the behavior will not simply go away on its own. Research suggests that sexual harassment behavior often continues escalate to more violent or intrusive behaviors on the part of the harasser as they become emboldened about getting away with the criminal behavior.

The initial step to take is to recognize the behavior for what it is— harassment. Remember the treatment one is receiving is unwanted whether it be sexual advances, comments, or a hostile work environment. Acknowledging and naming the circumstances or incident can be very difficult because the desire to engage in denial or minimizing what happened will be strong. Instead of ignoring what happened, be sure to acknowledge it to yourself and to your harasser. In other words, it is critical to let your harasser know immediately the first time the behavior occurs that you do not like it (e.g., that the sexual advances are unwanted or not reciprocated). This can happen by simply saying "no" or by shrugging off the hands of the harasser off your shoulder or other body parts. A body shiver can also be effective in showing that the attention is not desired. Another way to show your displeasure is to freeze in place if you were moving at the time of the comment or unwanted touching.

Avoid the temptation to laugh at risqué jokes or flirtatious comments. Under no circumstances should you join in the banter, start laughing, or give the impression of ambiguity. Of course, the path of least resistance would be to dish it back in a show of toughness or holding your own; however, this could muddy the waters. Likewise, be sure to avoid giving incongruent nonverbal cues by smiling, acting embarrassed, or offering direct eye contact when it happens. Another suggestion would include to avoid answering overly personal questions or those of a sexual nature by your harasser. Do not offer to do special favors for your harasser that extend outside of your role as a student or employee. Above all else, remember that if you maintain a calm and professional approach it is less likely you will be labeled as participating in the bullying behavior at school or your workplace. Although it is never appropriate to blame the victim for the sexual harassment by pointing to areas like dress, it is recommended that in a workplace, school, or public setting appropriate and professional attire be worn. Make sure that you are adhering to the cultural norms of dress or any stated expectations or policies about clothing (such as no flip flops).

More recently, Gretchen Carlson has created what she dubs a "twelve-point playbook" for when someone has been at the receiving end of sexual harassment. This guide includes steps or considerations for moving forward. The first step regardless of your environment refers to knowing your rights. If you are in a workplace, learn about what are the laws and be sure to read through the employee handbook. Make sure to read your contract if you have one. Many service jobs may not have a formal written contract, but be sure to read anything published or handed to you at your employee orientation. Many companies will have statements and keep in mind that sexual harassment is against the law. One challenge to pursuing claims of sexual harassment is employee status (e.g., paid vs. unpaid workers). For example, being an intern within a company in many states means a lack of protection under workplace law. This makes this category of workers who are already younger and newer to the company especially vulnerable. More recently, some states have passed laws to extend these protections within the workplace to interns, and bills have been brought forward by the U.S. House of Representatives, but it is important to consult local and state laws early in the process.

The need to document cannot be stressed enough. When one experiences inappropriate sexual advances or other inappropriate behavior, they need to keep track of specifics by writing it down. Be sure to document details around the date of an incident, people involved, locations, and names of witnesses. Each time something happens, it should be included in this journal. Do not make the false assumption that it was a one-time event that will go away on its own.

A strategy for documenting events is to send emails to your inbox and keep an electronic folder. Just make sure that your harasser does not have access to your written or electronic journaling. In addition to chronicling the events, be sure to gather any written proof such as sexually explicit texts or emails. Be sure to save voice mails and take pictures of anything offensive like signs or posters. If the attention is associated with a social media post, be sure to take a screenshot and save. If harassment occurs in a workplace, the person should save performance reviews if applicable. This may not be relevant for hourly employees or those in a service profession. Interns may not be subject to performance reviews. In an academic setting, be sure to track grades or relevant information about school performance.

31. What are the barriers to reporting sexual harassment? Why don't people report?

There are a myriad of reasons people fail to report sexual harassment when it has occurred in a school setting or workplace. Studies consistently demonstrate that only a small number (often well below 2 percent) of sexual harassment incidents are reported despite many individuals admitting to having experienced such behavior. Why are there so few complaints when sexual harassment is clearly happening?

One of the biggest reasons cited by victims relates to fearing retaliation resulting from their complaint. Whether real or imagined, there is a strong perception that things will become worse if sexual harassment is reported. At school, if a student reports bullying, they expect to experience even more negative and intense attention. If at a person's place of employment, it is anticipated that one can experience subtle discrimination, demotion, or even the loss of one's job. In other words, by reporting sexual harassment, the target gets caught in the crosshairs of receiving continued victimization as a direct consequence of speaking up. Many teenagers do not have the luxury of transferring to other schools. Missing classes or school directly impacts academic performance and can jeopardize a student's future aspirations. Speaking up at a person's place of work is also difficult when one does not have an easy way to make a shift to another job and would impact one's ability to secure a professional reference. Especially for teenagers in customer service jobs (such as fast-food restaurants and grocery stores), these jobs may represent the first step into the workplace and are not always readily available for younger aged employees. However, employees of any age can feel the sting associated with reporting sexual harassment. Fearing being alienated by one's coworkers is a real concern. There have been documented cases in which employees are bullied by colleagues after speaking up. In one circumstance, an employee who had reported sexual harassment found a skeleton at her workstation when she arrived for the day. Also, although victims of sexual harassment are encouraged to report incidents to the human resources department, there is the common perception that management will not act on complaints, so therefore it is pointless.

There are numerous factors related to lack of reporting. Some of the most popularly cited ones include the following: (1) ignorance regarding sexual harassment and the law, (2) confusion and emotions surrounding sexual harassment, (3) fear of not being believed by others, (4) fears around potential consequences of being a victim, and (5) concerns for others (including the person doing the harassing). A victim may worry about not being believed by others or experience judgment like being under a microscope. Moreover, a victim of sexual harassment may anticipate feeling humiliated by bringing attention to the issue. Sadly, many victims worry about being treated differently or poorly by others. Some may fear being alienated by their peers or colleagues, but other concerns stem from the deep-seated worry that retaliation will result in job loss, demotion, or damage to one's career.

As noted, a major reason that people neglect to report sexual harassment has to do with ignorance related to the law. In other words, many female students did not even know that offensive behavior was against the law or was considered sexual harassment especially if done in a joking manner. For employees, studies have shown that up to one-third did not realize that behaviors such as offensive jokes and showing images of a sexual nature constituted illegal harassment. It is important to point out that people doing the harassing, whether bullies at school or harassers at the workplace, also were not always aware that their lewd behavior was sexual harassment and that they were breaking the law. Clearly, more education is continually needed to help develop a broad understanding of what actions constitute sexual harassment. Related to ignorance about the law itself is a lack of understanding about what to do if someone experiences sexual harassment at school or at work. It may not feel safe to talk to one's parents, teacher, or principal, for example. If working for a family-owned business where everyone knows everyone, it might be difficult to report an incident in a private manner.

Being sexually harassed is an emotionally charged experience without a doubt. In addition to not realizing that sexual harassment is illegal and thus, against the law, feeling confusion about the incident is quite common. For many victims, there is a tendency to blame oneself and one's role in what happened or to second-guess behaviors leading up to sexually harassing behaviors. For example, a frequent response is for the victim to wonder whether they showed a cue that they were interested in a relationship or attracted in some way to the harasser. "Was I overly flirtatious? Did I ask for it or dress too provocatively?" The victim might think—did I give the wrong impression or offer too much eye contact? It confounds the situation when the harasser is someone that the victim knows well—a friend, coworker, a family friend, or one's supervisor. The victim might second-guess the incident and question whether they reciprocated interest or did not state "no" clearly enough or make it known that attention was unwanted. Bottom line is that victims often blame themselves and worry about overreacting, and this confusion can be a barrier to reporting the incident even when it is undeniable that sexual harassment has taken place.

Just as the victim blames themselves, it is unfortunate that there is a tendency for victim blaming and shaming to take place by others. There might be unwelcome attention from the media, one's coworkers, or family members. People may not understand what happened or might attribute the incident to the way the victim acted and dressed or their "reputation." It is common for victims to have concerns about how making a complaint will be received by others. "Will they believe me that sexual harassment has occurred?" Gretchen Carlson later wrote that she was skewered on social media by those who blamed her for what had happened and made nasty comments like "she's too old and ugly to be sexually harassed" and "she wishes she was attractive enough to be sexually harassed." Many sexual harassment cases have become widely public affairs, which may deter some victims who do not wish to be in the spotlight or vilified. Victims may be accused of lying for financial gain or attention or to hurt someone else. These cases may be one person's word against the others.

There is also concern around the humiliation of having one's sexual harassment incident becoming public. Given that the attention was unwanted, the idea of one's dirty laundry being aired for the world to see is extremely unappealing. Naturally many people would choose to avoid conflict altogether or pretend the incident never happened. Denial is powerful. The problem is that the sexual harassment will not go away, and the humiliation is likely to continue either way. It is literally a no-win situation. However, a victim may feel humiliated in a different way if the incident is reported. Victims are often subjected to name-calling, verbal insults, and vulgar language. They will have to relive the incident over and over again in great details with the lawyers and in court. Certainly, there is worry that one's reputation is at stake. Sharing the incident repeatedly is embarrassing and humiliating for the victim.

A perceived consequence of reporting sexual harassment relates to losing one's job or being denied promotion. One's career path may feel threatened, or how one is viewed by their colleagues could change based on the incident. These fears play a strong role in deterring victims from reporting the incident. This fear of retaliation is a major driver in preventing both women and men from speaking up. As previously stated, victims may not have the autonomy to find another school or job. There may be dire consequences for sharing what happened. Being ostracized by one's peers or colleagues is a real fear. Being the "whistleblower" is often synonymous with being viewed as the troublemaker. As the victim, one might question, "If she or he did not say anything when the same thing happened, why is it up to me?" It is really difficult to become the central focus in the gossip mill. Let's face it: There is nothing straightforward about having to call something out that has been happening a long time with no checks, balances, or consequences. There may even be a culture of acceptance around the bad behavior that includes a long line of victims and bullies. Furthermore, labeling this negative behavior by reporting sexual harassment might be judged by other students or one's coworkers as "tattling" or worse yet accused of "wanting it" or "asking for it [the unwanted sexual attention]." The victim's reputation is literally on the line, which is not fair given that the harasser is the one who committed the illegal acts.

Finally, concern for others can be a barrier to reporting sexual harassment. In an attempt to avoid conflict, victims also worry about the effects on others rather than taking care of themselves. The victims fear the impact on their own family if reporting sexual harassment undermines their career aspirations or threatens their position in the company. But illogically victims may also be concerned about the family of the harasser—what will my supervisor's wife feel? If I report this, will this hurt my supervisor's kids? Given that many harassers are familiar people in the lives of the victims—fellow students at the same school, friends, or coworkers of many years, it is not surprising that it is difficult to stand up to negative events that have happened. While there are many barriers to reporting (which explains the high tendency for under-reporting), it is vital that resources are available for victims of sexual harassment.

32. What resources are available for victims of sexual harassment?

When one becomes a victim of sexual harassment, it can be confusing to know where to go. If a person experiences sexual harassment, the first inclination may be to seek help from the human resources department. Unfortunately, they may not be the ideal step for helping a victim due to their allegiance with the company. Many communities provide free or reduced legal advice to residents who do not have the means to afford them. Some attorneys will agree to cut their fees if a victim is willing to work with a more junior attorney in their firm. Getting neutral and objective advice can aid a victim in determining whether their incident rises to the level of being reported and what steps to take.

For those in a university setting, there are a variety of resources available for victims of sexual harassment. Because sexual harassment fits the category of gender discrimination, an important resource is the office of Title IX. Each university is required to have an independent office (separate from human resources) that can field complaints from students, faculty, and staff related to sexual harassment, gender discrimination, and sexual assault. Persons can go to their individual campus's webpage and google "Title IX" to find the appropriate process for seeking consultation or filing a formal complaint. There are national regulations around what the process entails and the level of confidentiality that a victim can expect with respect to their report. Meeting with a Title IX officer will allow a victim to decide whether to move forward with a formal complaint.

College campuses often have resources for victims of rape and sexual assault. These would be a good place to contact if one is a victim of sexual harassment. Centers of gender studies can be another resource at universities to seek support for gender discrimination or harassment over one's gender identity or sexual orientation. These support services will actively work to protect the confidentiality of victims.

If one is in high school or middle school, gender discrimination is still prohibited under Title IX laws. At one's school, it is expected for the school counselors to be equipped with the knowledge to help victims of sexual abuse, harassment, and assault. Even if this person does not treat the victims directly, the counselor can provide the necessary referrals to an appropriate mental health provider, support group, and other resources.

Likewise, at one's place of employment, depending on the size of the agency or company, there will be procedures and policies explaining what behaviors are not allowable as well as the appropriate actions to take if someone has fallen victim to sexual harassment. It is common for workplace settings to offer what is called EAP or Employee Assistance Program. EAP refers to interventions or support services that are made available to employees who are struggling with personal issues that directly relate to their work performance.

In addition to resources that are affiliated with one's school, employer, or community, there are numerous websites available for victims of sexual harassment. Many organizations have been founded, such as RAINN, to help individuals who have suffered from abuse, harassment, and assault to stand up to their perpetrators. Specifically, RAINN offers a hotline to direct individuals in need to the services in their area. Options for assistance may include free or reduced cost for legal services or treatment providers who specialize in trauma and sexual abuse. Support groups may be available for individuals who suffer from sexual assault, rape, and abuse. This may be helpful for providing immediate support from others who have experienced similar trauma and can validate feelings. A long list of specific resources including books, websites, and organizations are available in the back of this publication in the section entitled "Directory of Resources."

33. What support groups are available to help people who have been victims of sexual harassment?

The momentum of support groups as a tool to promote self-help was popularized in the 1970s with a mental health movement. Although self-help support groups popped up for individuals afflicted by a variety of struggles, the concept of peer support harkens back to the 1800s in psychiatric hospitals. Having the opportunity for encouragement from peers and staff was viewed as a positive and humane way to treat patients who suffered from mental illness and had been treated as outcasts by society. This different way of approaching the most ill patients was beneficial in the prognosis of even the most difficult cases.

Mental health professionals generally see the value in group-based therapy. Groups allow for socialization and the public acknowledgment of one's struggles, which can be a sign of tremendous personal growth.

While support groups are not always considered therapy, there is still an opportunity to connect with others and to acknowledge challenges and "slips" in the case of individuals recovering from addiction.

Support groups may be online or in-person experiences and meet for a variety of causes. Generally, support groups are distinct from group therapy in that they may be facilitated by the victims themselves or by a volunteer therapist. Support group meetings may take place in a church or other community center similarly to Alcoholics Anonymous. Membership and participation in these groups is free of charge (which is a definite bonus) and may have differing frequency depending on the group's or individual's preference. Support group members should allow for time to share stories and not interrupt one another.

Confidentiality is an absolute necessity for creating a safe space for victims to receive support for one another. Although a victim can search for resources within their community for active groups, social media has a plethora of Facebook groups as well for virtual support without needing to leave one's home. Feeling anonymous has been cited as a benefit of online support groups, but some individuals will prefer having an in-person experience.

The biggest benefit of participating in a support group regardless of the delivery format is the feeling of validation that comes from a shared experience. Victims have the chance to meet other victims and understand that they are not alone. The complex emotions—guilt, anger toward perpetrator, and shame—are expressed by others in the group and normalized. While the group does not replace the likely need for ongoing therapy with a licensed professional, having supportive members can help the victim along in the healing process. It is important not to feel isolated or alone in this extremely challenging time.

Referrals for active support groups might be offered by school counselors, trained therapists who work in this area, or attorneys who specialize in sexual harassment cases. In some cases, employers may have lists of resources. Finally, organizations like RAINN may have tips about local services that maintain up-to-date offerings of support groups in your area if you call their hotline.

34. How can therapy help victims of sexual harassment?

The negative consequences associated with experiencing sexual harassment and other forms of gender discrimination are widespread and can affect one throughout their life. Sexual harassment is unwanted like other forms of abuse, the victims are highly secretive and the scars are invisible. It is not an accident that prevalence rates of sexual harassment are much lower than the expected rate of occurrence. When someone is a victim of sexual harassment, they will likely experience a myriad of emotions and reactions to the incident.

There may be guilt and blaming of oneself for the incident along with questioning whether one invited the attention. It is quite possible that one feels pressured to speak up or report the incident but fears the repercussions for doing so. In fact, if the victim is in a culture that actively accepts or condones sexual harassment and gender discrimination, they may feel helpless and hopeless. Therefore, seeking treatment in the form of mental health therapy is essential to moving past the incident and coming to peace with one's situation. Perhaps one decides not to report the incident but is still able to express negative emotions and resolution. Or alternatively, maybe one works through therapy and is empowered to submit a complaint against one harasser. They have received and can continue to receive the necessary support from a professional treatment provider. Why is it so helpful to have a trained clinician rather than a family or friend? This person can provide an unbiased view of the situation and will maintain confidentiality as an ethical obligation of their job. A victim will not become the topic of gossip when working with a therapist like it could happen if one's "friend" spills the beans. Although therapists can just be there to listen, they have been trained to help victims find their own solutions and path to peace.

It is important for victims of trauma and abuse to seek the help and support they need with the recognition that healing will not happen automatically by pressing a switch. Like any traumatic experience, triggers can creep up when one is least expecting them to occur. Therapy allows for a safe and confidential place to express what happened to a trained professional. That trained professional will not only be an active listener but will ask the right questions to encourage the client to delve deeper in expressing mixed emotions about the incident.

There is no standard protocol for seeking treatment other than needing the courage to share what has happened with a stranger. However, trained counselors will listen without judgment, and they offer a safe place to the victim to get angry or express whatever emotion is triggered. There is an opportunity for validation of what has occurred and the reinforcement that being sexually harassed is not their fault. Helping to dissuade a victim from accepting blame for being harassed is key, as well as flushing out the complicated web of feelings that surround the sexual harassment behaviors. Affirmation of these feelings and complex emotions helps to normalize them. The trained clinician will likely use therapeutic statements such as "I can see you are really hurting right now" as opposed to trying to solve the problem or questioning one's feelings, reaction to the harassment, or behaviors. Flexibility will also be emphasized by the trained counselor, and treatment is all about going where the client wants to go and needs to go. Each client is treated as unique and has one's own path for healing.

It is important to acknowledge that an event such as sexual harassment or bullying at school might influence one's mood or increase the likelihood of depression or anxiety. Therefore, the trained counselor can help provide appropriate referrals for psychiatrists to receive additional support and medications if needed in addition to the treatment for those symptoms. The biggest benefit of receiving treatment in the form of mental health counseling is the continued validation and reassurance during a turbulent time. The victim may be judged by others at their school and receive negative attention from the other party. Having positive support will be critical during this difficult time.

35. What is the best way to help someone who may have been a victim of sexual harassment?

While there are clear steps that a bystander can take when they witness sexual harassment, it might be less straightforward to know how to help another student or coworker who has experienced sexually harassing behaviors or bullying. It can be a bit intimidating of course, but the good news is that most schools and places of employment have outlined specific policies and procedures about how to handle sexual harassment. You may not know the ins and outs at your school, but if you suspect another student has suffered from sexual harassment you can still act. Firstly, remember that you will want to express your concerns to a teacher, school counselor, or trusted adult. Be sure to be explicit about any changes you have noticed in your fellow student's mood, behaviors, or health status.

If you feel comfortable doing so, there is nothing more powerful than expressing your concerns directly to your student (or coworker). The best way to create a receptive communication is to use "I" statements as they are more effective than saying "you" statements that can put someone on the spot. For example, one can say something like "I am concerned because it seems like you haven't been your cheerful self lately." When preparing for the conversation, it is a good idea to have some resources at your fingertips like the RAINN website and any local services that can help the person you suspect has been the victim of sexual harassment. You can offer to walk the student to the school counselor or nurse's office for support. Additionally, you can share the hotline number or even help make the phone call to the RAINN organization to determine free services in the area.

With respect to a place of employment, your role of potential support may be different if you are a coworker versus the manager or direct supervisor of the person you suspect has been sexually harassed. As a supervisor, if an employee comes forward with a sexual harassment complaint there is an obligation to act. Hopefully, regardless of your role in the organization you can be there as a person who takes time to listen without judgment to what has happened. As the supervisor, there will be the need to document the conversation and to take the information to human resources.

If an employee does not come forward to report an incident but you suspect that sexual harassment has occurred, there is still responsibility to act. As a coworker, you might report to a trusted supervisor or bring your concerns directly to your colleague. Although the conversation may feel uncomfortable, the supervisor or coworker might express concern about the noticed changes. These may include but not be limited to the following: missing work, shifting clothing choices to ultraconservative dress attire, hearing rumors in the office, noticing discomfort of the employee around certain individuals, observing a withdrawal from social interactions, or a sudden unwillingness to participate in social functions (e.g., lunch). It is necessary to be familiar with the policies or ask about them. Supervisors should be positive role models of respect and civility in the office and should monitor their own behaviors and biases that may lead to discriminatory practices. Finally, a safe environment should be created at the workplace or school so that the person who has been the victim of sexual harassment comes forward voluntarily to report the incident.

36. What is bystander intervention? What should I do when I witness sexual harassment?

Both sexual harassment and bullying are common occurrences within school settings that are unfortunately associated with numerous psychological and physical consequences for the victim. Regardless of whether bullying takes place in person or involves what has been labeled as "electronic aggression" (otherwise referred to or involving cyber bullying), the potential for harm is extensive and can target both middle school and high school students alike. It is well known that most students (up to 80 percent or more) report being exposed to victimization of peers in the form of bullying or sexual harassment within their school. Approximately 30 percent of students (across middle school and high school) admit to bullying others or being the target of bullying behavior, whereas 40–84 percent report having been the victim of sexual harassment. Moreover, 40 percent of middle school students had observed sexual harassment take place in their school. This high prevalence of observing both bullying and sexual harassment suggests that there are often witnesses for these acts of peer aggression. Therefore, the role of bystander intervention is critical for prevention of bullying and for addressing sexual harassment in schools and other contexts. Responses by the bystanders or witnesses can be varied and multifold.

Firstly, the bystander may opt to join in on the aggressive act. This unfortunate response results in having the witness reinforce the bad behavior by assisting the bully, which can escalate violence and negative consequences for the victim. The second potential reaction of a bystander is for the witness to defend the victim. If the witness elects for this response, the person becomes an active bystander. The active bystander represents a defender of the victim, who might actively halt the aggression or intervene by calling out to the bully to stop or physically pulling the bully away from the victim. Another possibility is for the active bystander to immediately report the incident, go to locate help, or to seek assistance from a teacher or adult. Being an active bystander could involve recording the event for documentation. An active bystander may also help by supporting the student who was victimized by consoling them or taking their side. In addition to joining in the victimization or being a defender, another possible response involves ignoring the incident by looking away or walking by without doing anything. This form of a response by a witness is considered inaction and is not helpful for addressing bullying or sexual harassment.

Although most incidents of sexual harassment and bullying involve witnesses so that the bully has an audience to show their power and control, people rarely intervene to help the victim. In fact, bystanders assist less than 20 percent of the time. This lack of action, response, or intervention is less about supporting the perpetrator or due to lack of interest and more about feeling powerless or lacking confidence about how to help or intervene.

The behavior of bystanders has been studied by social psychologists for decades. An early study attempted to understand why people had failed to act when they were in the presence of a murder that took place in 1964. Research has demonstrated that several factors are at work when bystanders do not intervene. One huge barrier to acting or intervening is related to the bystander's perception of whether incident is an emergency. When the situation is not seen as critical or serious, the witness fails to act. Another factor that prevents intervention involves the diffusion of responsibility that occurs in the presence of other witnesses. In other words, the tendency to intervene is vastly reduced when bystanders hold the belief that other students will help the victim. Thus, the presence of other peers inhibits one's own sense of responsibility and no one acts to help. Researchers have confirmed that this failure to act in a group versus individual setting might be tied to fear of being embarrassed in front of one's peers when there is an audience.

Examining the bystander effect is important for considering bullying prevention in schools. Witnesses should view the incident as an emergency and assume there is a need to act regardless of the response (or potential inaction) of other bystanders who may be present. A bystander should take steps to identify the optimal way to reduce or halt aggression and to assist the victim. Depending on the size of the bully and bystander, the best course of action may be calling or texting for help. Recording the incident or agreeing to serve as a physical witness can be helpful to the target of sexual harassment whether the behavior takes place at school, off campus, or at work. While the victim may decide against making a formal complaint, when someone acknowledges that a wrong act has occurred it is powerful and validating. Finally, the power of standing up for someone else is undeniable. Having a bystander tell the bully to "knock it off" takes a lot of courage but might make the difference in the quality of life for another human being. Consoling a victim after the incident is helpful as well to prevent feelings of hopelessness, being alone, and experiencing social isolation. Telling a parent, teacher, or trusted adult is important so that you do not have to face this challenging situation alone or find yourself the victim of retaliation. Observing aggression can be troubling, and you may need to process your feelings and emotions. Schools should raise awareness about sexual harassment and bullying by educating students the role that bystanders can take to intervene when they witness an incident take place.

37. How can sexual harassment be prevented at schools? What educational strategies can be adopted?

The first step for prevention within schools is to acknowledge that sexual harassment and bullying are a problem. If a school identifies sexual harassment prevention as a problem and a priority, they need to commit to invest in strategies to institute change. Sounds like a tall order, doesn't it? Yes, for schools a comprehensive approach is needed when addressing and preventing sexual harassment and bullying. It is insufficient to merely talk about getting rid of bullying to change behavior. The level of tolerance for any unacceptable behaviors must be zero, and swift action must be taken when bullying does occur. Furthermore, students must be made to feel safe to intervene as bystanders or to report incidents if they fall victim to bullying or sexual harassment. There should be clear steps for a victim or bystander to take if they witness or experience sexual harassment on school premises, off campus, or on social media. For sustainable prevention, infrastructure must be put in place that goes beyond a one-off initiative, program, or event to provide training, manage complaints, and support victims.

In recent decades, policies and procedures have been formalized, and Title IX coordinators have been appointed to field complaints within school settings. However, for prevention to truly occur and for cases to decrease, the cultural norms of acceptable behavior must shift so that bullying is not tolerated on any level. That is, teachers, administrators, students, and parents should receive education to raise awareness about sexual harassment as well as bystander intervention training. Moreover, school counselors and nurses who represent the "front line" for complaints should have additional specialized knowledge about how to best support victims of sexual harassment.

Bullying prevention programs are increasingly common in middle and high schools. Effective modules include scenarios to depict different forms of peer aggression to bring it to life. In addition, role plays about how to intervene or stand up to the bully are recommended. Parents and the broader community represent key allies and should receive education geared to stop sexual harassment and bullying outside of the school. Parents should be taught about how to discourage bullying and aggressive behavior at home as well as how to serve as positive role models. Parents can participate in workshops, discussion groups, or programs that include parent and child dyads.

Teachers play a vital role in eliminating gender bias in the classroom at an early age. Elementary school teachers should monitor their own biases and language around gender and other social categories (e.g., body size, race). They should assign gender-neutral tasks to their students and avoid reinforcing stereotypes in their comments. Middle school teachers can expand curricula to be more inclusive of the diverse ways that women have historically contributed to society. Middle and high school students can learn about sexism and how to support each other to reduce sexual harassment in school. Social studies or health classes can cover topics such as what is sexual harassment, the consequences of bullying, and the steps to take if one is a victim or bystander.

38. How can I get involved in the cause to raise awareness about sexual harassment?

Although awareness about sexual harassment has improved with the introduction of Title IX laws against gender discrimination, very public court cases, and the #MeToo movement, there is much more that remains to be done. On the personal level, every one of us has the obligation to speak out against sexual harassment when it occurs. No matter one's age or gender, we might be a bystander (or witness) to an incident in which sexual harassment takes place. It is important to remember that speaking up may happen in different forms. For example, it may not be safe to confront the harasser in the moment, but one can talk to a trusted adult, teacher, coworker, or friend. It is important to discuss the experience as a victim or a bystander as close to the incident as possible so that as many details can be provided. If one waits to discuss what has taken place, they might lose their nerve or get distracted with other life responsibilities, and the opportunity to bring awareness to the issue is lost.

If you are interested in raising awareness about sexual harassment, there are also several more formal ways you can jump in. The national organization, RAINN, offers plenty of ways for people to get involved in the cause of sexual harassment. April is Sexual Assault Awareness and Prevention month each year with different themes and activities geared toward increasing awareness around the topic. Volunteers can share resources and statistics with others on their own social media. RAINN has also shared some ways that friends and family members can provide support to survivors of sexual harassment. There is a toolkit so that people know the right things to say to be supportive and listen without judgment.

Whether with RAINN, another organization, or at a local level, one can get involved with or organize events related to sexual harassment awareness. Students or teachers can bring in speakers during the year or into health classes. Professional development opportunities or events can be organized to discuss the topic and how to address sexual harassment in schools and the workplace.

At the local level, you might choose to act to serve as an advocate for survivors. As an advocate, you can make sure that your school or work-place has policies in place that protect against gender discrimination and sexual harassment. Perhaps you can lead an effort to introduce bystander intervention training at your school to raise awareness about sexual harassment and how to halt peer aggression. This training may include ways to "call out" gender discrimination or sexual harassment when you see it taking place. You can participate or organize a march, protest, or write an opinion article to your local newspaper.

You can be a trusted friend or support for someone who is a survivor of sexual harassment or abuse. Nothing is more valuable than having a loyal and confidential support. If you are a survivor yourself, you may feel inclined to speak up and make some noise about sexual harassment. Make sure that you are in a place that is safe for you to share your story with others. The more you can get the word out there, the more that people will understand real-life examples of what should not happen in schools or in the workplace. Perhaps you can organize a panel discussion with trained clinicians in the area to share the steps to take if someone has been a victim of sexual harassment, your recovery story, and the resources in the area.

Another way to get involved in helping the cause of sexual harassment is to begin or advocate for the creation of a support group. Regardless of whether you organize a support group that meets at a local church or community center as opposed to an online Facebook group, having the connection to other survivors is powerful and helpful.

39. How can individuals help build a culture of respect at workplaces to prevent sexual harassment?

Although it is easy to assume that adults know better than to bully one another, workplaces have often been the site of sexual harassment. There-fore, in the interest of developing a culture of civility that does not allow room for sexual harassment, it is crucial for the employer to take several prescribed steps for preventing undesirable behaviors. Many companies in the past couple of decades have adopted strict policies prohibiting sex-ual harassment following lawsuits in the 1980s and 1990s; however, some of the smaller businesses have less well-defined and publicized guidelines and procedures.

In order to impact the work culture, the employer must get the buy-in of employees and set the tone for clear expectations. In particular, anti-harassment policies must be specific and should involve the following: a legal definition of sexual harassment adapted from EEOC; description of behaviors to be avoided in the workplace; steps to take if someone falls victim to bullying, sexual harassment, or discrimination of any kind; who will field complaints and how to contact them; how any complaints will be handled; and what disciplinary actions will take place. Disciplinary actions will likely involve termination, which should be spelled out. Furthermore, the policy should be provided in writing to all employees when they begin employment and should be discussed during orientation. There should be clear support from the top and the management, which might come in the form of a small presentation during orientation that makes it clear that sexual harassment is taken seriously, creates a hostile work environment, is a human rights issue, is not tolerated, and will result in disciplinary action.

Being able to bring attention to a situation in which you personally felt uncomfortable (as a potential victim of sexual harassment, workplace bullying, or gender discrimination) helps others realize the unintended consequences of their actions. If you have the courage to speak up, hearing your story will help personalize the face of sexual harassment for those in the workplace who may not take it seriously. In some cases, sexual harassment happens in the context of making a joke, but it is no laughing matter. Helping others develop empathy for the victim is key if you feel comfortable allowing yourself to be vulnerable. Scheduling one-on-one meetings helps make these conversations a little more effective with potential allies in your organization.

Secondarily, it may also empower others to intervene if they are bystanders. The author of this book recently found herself in a meeting where she felt uncomfortable with the use of sexist language related to a potential hiring action. The words, "We can hire a guy who can bring his grant" did not sit well with her. She was the only one in the meeting with nine other men. Her boss did not speak up nor did the others in higher ranking positions. She found herself feeling shrinking and experiencing disengagement. After the Zoom meeting, she was frustrated for not saying anything. But she followed up on her discomfort by meeting with several other attendees in the meeting. They not only listened and empathized with her experience in the meeting but also committed to saying something if it happened again. The importance of educating and bringing situations up helps increase the potential for bystander intervention.

Educating all members of the workforce is the most effective way to ensure that there are clear expectations about conduct and acceptable (as well as unacceptable) behaviors. It is helpful to use specific scenarios to make sexual harassment "real" to employees and to show examples. While conducting training, it is prudent to have employees sign a pledge of workplace civility that represents their commitment to abiding by the policies set forth. A pledge helps to underscore the priority of an organization to eliminate harassment, bullying, and discrimination from the workplace.

Sexual Harassment and Popular Culture

40. What role does the media play in the development of a culture of sexual harassment?

Media's role in shaping culture has been examined across evolving trends including social norms. The way that one's gender is portrayed in movies and in television ads, for example, can build one's conscience about what a man or woman is supposed to do. In other words, gender discrimination and sexualizing females can become normalized and even accepted by one's culture when the pattern plays out repeatedly in a variety of media outlets (magazines, television, movies). The movie 9 *to* 5 immediately comes to mind when thinking about sexual harassment. In this popular movie from the 1980s, the stereotypical office culture is depicted by a male supervisor who orders around female subordinates, who are ridiculed and subjected to sexually inappropriate behavior. Although the movie falls in the comedy genre, the negative effects are brought to light with a spotlight shining on the inequity and power dynamics present in the workplace.

Likewise, the media has acted as a vehicle to keep women focused on constantly striving to be more beautiful and attractive for their predictably male love interests. These images not only serve to objectify and sexualize women and trivialize their skills beyond appearance but also are narrowly focused, heterosexist (assume male and female attraction), and biased against those who fall outside of the gender binary.

The media takes a deeply personal event that is private and humiliating and shines a light on it. The 2019 film *Bombshell* clearly depicts how media can play a role in making sexual harassment a public event. In the movie based on real events, Gretchen Carlson's experience with Fox News CEO Roger Ailes is documented. Other women, such as Megyn Kelly, are shown to come forward to support Gretchen's claim, but the film demonstrates the impact of lodging a complaint on the victim. Suddenly Gretchen (and Megyn) find that they are the news story. The effect is to be thrust in the media spotlight and to become the target of haters on social media and beyond.

In Gretchen Carlson's book *Be Fierce: Stop Harassment and Take Your Power Back*, she describes how, after enduring years of sexual harassment from Roger Ailes, she faced immense cyberbullying and mean tweets from people who did not even know her. These critics accused Gretchen of being "old and washed up" and accused her of seeking attention for a career on a downward trajectory. In fact, the negative press that victims experience is sometimes said to be worse than the sexual harassment itself. This unfortunate reality explains why so few individuals report sexual harassment or move forward to make a formal claim. In addressing sexual harassment associated with a person who possesses a powerful position within a company, it takes money, time, and persistence. The victim will likely be dragged through the mud and may suffer both in the short term and the long term in their careers. In sum, the media amplifies the claim—it thrusts both the accused and the accuser in the spotlight.

41. What role do sports play in the development of a culture that permits sexual harassment?

There is strong evidence that cultures that tend to perpetuate traditional gender roles and stereotypes may be more likely to breed a variety of power dynamics such as hazing and sexual harassment. Sports, for instance, have been identified as a culture that objectifies girls and women and has historically been accepting of sexually explicit and derogatory comments about females. This gender discrimination has played out a variety of ways both formally and informally and has gone unchallenged. There are clear examples of sexual assault and rape that have been unfortunately associated with sport teams such as the 2006 forcible rape charges brought against the Duke Lacrosse players. Sexual harassment has been more difficult to prove in sports, like it has been in school, military, and work settings. However, there is some evidence that behaviors that constitute sexual harassment are widespread.

An example of sexual harassment is when a head coach makes unwanted advances to someone on the coaching staff or sport medicine personnel. Sexual harassment could also include comments made by a coach or athletic trainer about an athlete's appearance. While they are widely known to exist, an athlete is unlikely to report due to the power dynamic associated with their sport career and possibly a scholarship on the line. Instead, the athlete might endure the negative behaviors during their time on the team with no consequences to the perpetrator. Incidents of young athletes in elite gymnastics and figure skating experiencing a number of damaging behaviors were documented in the 1996 book by author Joan Ryan called *Little Girls in Pretty Boxes: The Making and Breaking of Elite Gymnasts and Figure Skaters*.

Having a sport culture that breeds sexual harassment is not limited to athletes or junior coaches as victims. Recently, 15 employees of the Washington Redskins (now renamed the Washington Football Team) came forward with sexual harassment claims. This alleged sexual harassment exemplifies the way that the culture of sport can perpetuate sexual harassment for many years. Women indicated that they were encouraged to wear revealing clothing such as low-cut blouses and skirts as well as told to flirt with clients. Furthermore, they were subjected to verbal sexual harassment by their male colleagues in the form of explicit and berating comments about their appearance. Women throughout the organization revealed being told by veteran female colleagues to avoid open stairways for fear of having men in the organization look up their skirts. Still other female employees reported receiving sexually explicit texts from male colleagues within the football team's organization. In addition to creating a hostile work environment by making women within the environment extremely uncomfortable, these women described how their dream career in pro sports was undermined. They expressed feeling decreased motivation to pursue their aspirations and experienced decreased morale when experiencing sexual harassment in a structure without support in place to handle complaints. While this incident thrust the Washington Football Team into the spotlight, it is expected that the culture of sport that uplifts masculinity may function as a likely place for sexual harassment to occur without being challenged. In fact, the *Journal of Clinical Sport Psychology* published a special issue for their journal in 2019 that exposed sexual harassment at all competitive levels of sport.

One of the bright spots in sport has been Troy Vincent, who serves as the executive vice president of the NFL football operations and who has played for the league himself. He has shared his childhood experiences of witnessing domestic violence and has spoken out against sexual harassment and assault in the sport culture. He advocates for bystander intervention training and for taking tangible steps for prevention of sexual harassment.

42. Which famous people/celebrities have reported sexual harassment?

Sexual harassment has occurred for decades and for many years did not have a name or consequence. Powerful institutions like Hollywood had an age-old reputation of having the "casting couch." There was the unspoken understanding that female and male actors would suffer both harassment and assault as part of the casting call. There was little or no legal protection for these actresses and actors who operated as free agents without the Title VII protection of the Civil Rights Act. When the *New York Times* breaking story exposed years of abuse on the part of Harvey Weinstein who was a movie mogul, it became clear that even "big name" celebrities were not immune from his destructive behavior. Both actresses and employees were subjected to unwanted sexual advances that constituted both harassment and assault on the part of Harvey Weinstein. While there were numerous victims, some of the celebrities stepped out to give a face to sexual harassment.

Significantly, Alyssa Milano used her Twitter account to encourage those who had suffered from sexual harassment to respond with a hashtag and the words "me too" on their feed. She herself reported suffering sexual harassment. In addition to Milano, Ashley Judd, Gwyneth Paltrow, Uma Thurman, Jennifer Lawrence, and Angelina Jolie were super celebrities when they decided to speak out and publicly come forward as part of the momentum for #MeToo movement that was accelerated. Other celebrities included but are not limited to Lady Gaga, American singer-songwriter, and Viola Davis, American actress and producer.

In 2018, Christine Blasey Ford, a respected attorney, came into the spotlight with an incredibly public hearing for providing credible testimony related to the Supreme Court nominee, Brett Kavanaugh, of inappropriate sexual behavior while they were in college. The Senate vote of 50-48 confirmed Kavanaugh's appointment but exposed a horrendously common experience for college coeds.

The film *Bombshell* was released in 2019 and showcased years of sexual harassment among female employees of Fox News. Well-known news anchors such as Gretchen and Megyn Kelly were thrust into the public spotlight as they became the news story for reporting about what had happened to them. CEO Roger Ailes had sexually harassed women for years, and his inappropriate advances were documented.

43. What is the #MeToo movement? What sparked this movement?

The #MeToo movement represents the single largest social movement to bring awareness and attention to the issue of sexual harassment. Unlike other progress made to address gender discrimination and sexual harassment, this momentum did not result in reaction to a courtroom ruling, but it was rather on social media with the general public. The "#" (hashtag) has become the social media way to mark and categorize conversation threads. With the emergence of #MeToo, the social media became the platform to acknowledge one's own victimization. In fact, the author of this book realized her own victimization had taken place over 25 years prior due to the awareness associated with the #MeToo movement. It had been buried in the deep recesses of her memory, but it was brought to light and she acknowledged to herself and others on social media with the single post of "me too."

While often victims of sexual harassment are traditionally secretive and often go unreported, this call to post "me too" allowed a way for individuals of all ages, race/ethnic groups, genders, and socioeconomic status to give voice to their experience (no matter how long ago it occurred). Women who participated, regardless of whether only by typing the two words or by elaborating about their experience, reported feeling supported by others on social media and empowered for coming out of the dark.

Sexual harassment has been reported across the globe and continues to occur even during times when society is thought to value being politically correct. Certainly, awareness of this problem has increased with high-profile politicians and celebrities being accused and found guilty of committing sexual harassment. Interestingly, Tarana Burke, a Black civil rights activist, began using the term "Me Too" to raise awareness about sexual harassment back in 2006. Specifically, Burke, a survivor herself, leveraged the social media platform of MySpace to post a tweet on her account with the phrase intended to induce solidarity and validation that comes from a shared experience of survival.

There was a delay in public outcry of support that resulted from social-ized expectations of gender at work, school, and in society. The #MeToo movement became mainstream in 2017 to bring attention to the wide-spread prevalence of sexual harassment and sexual assault against women (and the author) in the workplace. The phrase #MeToo was amplified and given an additional platform when Alyssa Milano, an actress in the United States with many followers, posted on her Twitter account on October 15 with a request for people to hashtag and type "me too" in their status if they had ever been sexually harassed or assaulted.

Numerous other high-profile female celebrities tweeted about their per-sonal experience, which led to a powerful realization that sexual harass-ment is pervasive in the entertainment field. However, perhaps more noteworthy was the number of women who responded within 24 hours from all different professions and occupations—doctors, nurses, teachers, lawyers, and many more. This movement that started as an informal post-ing of a hashtag via social media has spanned to become a large effort to identify wrongdoing as well as to enforce and strengthen laws within the United States and around the world.

44. How is "Time's Up" the next step in the #MeToo movement?

If #MeToo movement represents the largest movement associated with sexual harassment, the Time's Up movement can surely be credited as the sequel that kept the conversation going. While the #MeToo movement received more attention due to participation by well-known celebrities, the movement was broadly represented by diverse voices. Victims of all ages, genders, and occupations and from various socioeconomic status levels were part of this movement. By contrast, the Time's Up movement was really limited to what is often referred to the "top 1 percent."

The Time's Up movement was instigated by celebrities in Hollywood and others with financial means one year after the #MeToo movement. #MeToo was prompted by Alyssa Milano's tweet on social media encour-aging those who had been sexually harassed or assaulted to post "me too" in their status. Celebrities and other victims posted in response to sexual harassment cases such as Harvey Weinstein.

In November 2017, the Alianza Nacional de Campesinas wrote a letter to show solidarity with these celebrities on behalf of over 700,000 women who worked in farms throughout the United States. Several initiatives were spurred from that response, including the following: (1) call to wear black at the 75th Golden Globe Awards on the red carpet; (2) establish a legal defense fund to support victims of sexual harassment; (3) advocate for legislation to punish perpetrators for sexual harassment; and (4) establish gender parity within talent agencies.

Many women and men wore black at that event and others throughout the year. They used their microphones to speak out about injustices related to sexual harassment and assault. Well-known singers Cindy Lauper, Kesha, and Lady Gaga wore all-black outfits or white roses to the Grammys to show support for the "Time's Up" movement, and many speeches were delivered to bring attention to the widespread issue.

This movement was highly successful in raising money (over $22 million to date) for a legal defense fund founded by lawyer Roberta Kaplan to fight sexual harassment and sexual assault cases in the workplace. The movement was also effective in advocating for strict legislation to penalize companies that turn a blind eye to ongoing and reported sexual harassment. Moreover, the Time's Up movement was able to sign up hundreds of attorneys to help fight these cases on a volunteer basis.

Case Studies

The following case studies are intended to provide "real-life" examples of how sexual harassment can present itself in a variety of situations. In this section of the book, there are five scenarios that depict different case examples. Each case illustration will describe the details of a fictionalized account of sexual harassment as well as provide the recommended actions and plan to address the problem.

1. PHOEBE IS HARASSED IN EIGHTH GRADE

Phoebe is a 13-year-old shy girl from a small town in Colorado. She has started eighth grade after her family moved to North Carolina. It is quite a culture shock along with the humidity and the Southern accent. Sometimes it seems like a whole different language with expressions that make her feel like an outsider. Being a loner by nature, she had enjoyed Colorado because it offered hiking and skiing, where she could blow off steam and spend time in nature. Despite the changes she experiences, Phoebe has finally made a few friends and is getting used to her academic coursework. Her teachers have worked with her to make sure she is up to speed on the lessons.

Some of the boys in her grade are real jokesters whose sole mission is to terrorize their female classmates. Being in classes is okay, but Phoebe feels stressed out every time she must change classrooms throughout the day and constantly looks over her shoulder when she goes to her locker. There are two boys, Kenny and Rick, who think it is funny to come over on either side of her, grab her pants or skirt, and pull it down to her ankles. It is not uncommon when they come from behind her that her underwear also slides down in the process, leading to extreme embarrassment.

While Phoebe knows that she is not the only girl in her grade who is experiencing this behavior from the mean boys, she is especially sensitive to the fact that she is the new kid in school. It feels like she is being bullied because she is an easy target. She does not want to be mean to the boys, but she is sick of the humiliation she feels when it happens to her. Phoebe tries to play defense by wearing bun-huggers (track shorts) or bicycling shorts under her clothing, but their pranks continue. Out of frustration, Phoebe shares what is happening at school with her mother. They go together to visit with the principal about the issue. Principal Brown responds by saying, "This is the way that boys show that they like a girl in eighth grade. She should be flattered to be receiving the attention." Unfortunately, this apathy toward incidences that scream of sexual harassment does not help resolve the situation or validate how Phoebe is feeling.

After receiving a dissatisfactory response from the school's administration, Phoebe becomes highly discouraged and starts on a downward spiral. She begins to experience anxiety during classes and her grades start suffering. Her motivation to do well in school diminishes, and she lacks the passion to put time and energy into assignments. She misses school due to feeling ill but suspects that her sickness might be tied to her continuous state of stress. She develops severe depression and begins to self-harm in private. Sadly, she finds comfort from inflicting pain by cutting her arms and legs in areas that she can cover with clothing. Her mother discovers this self-harming behavior when she goes into Phoebe's room unannounced. What should she do to get Phoebe the help she needs?

Analysis

Phoebe's situation clearly fits the definition of sexual harassment within the K-12 school setting. Unfortunately, school administrators should be the ones to protect students from bullying and other types of harassment and abuse, but this was not the outcome for this fictitious eighth grader, even after she and her mother brought the issue to Mr. Brown's awareness.

This case illustration has similarities with a case that occurred in the state of Minnesota several decades ago. While the principal in the real-life situation reacted in a consistent fashion by chalking up a particular boy's unwanted behavior as flirting, the case took a legal turn. The student and one of her classmates appealed to and testified to the Minnesota legislature about the ongoing sexual harassment being experienced at their junior high school. Unfortunately, the problems did not end there. Following the girls' brave testimony to the state legislature, one of the members in the state legislature in the Minnesota case was reluctant to act for the fear of tarnishing the principal's reputation and seemed unconcerned about the actual bullying and effects on the victims. A transcription of the student's testimony was shared with the school, who accused her of lying when she testified. As one would imagine, the stress that this placed on the student and her family was tremendous.

Finally, in 1989 a comprehensive sexual violence bill was passed by the Minnesota state legislature. This bill moved the needle to require all K-12 schools to have a sexual harassment policy in place and to take action in a number of ways. This means that students who face harassment like Phoebe can report what they are experiencing and should expect results from the school administrators. Otherwise they have every right to press charges and may receive damages.

In the original case in Minnesota, the Minnesota Department of Human Rights determined that the school did not appropriately deal with the reports of sexual harassment. Given that the school failed to act in a timely fashion, they were liable and found to contribute to an environment that in fact "promoted sexual harassment." This student ended up settling out of court and received $40,000 in damages.

More importantly, Phoebe's case highlighted some common psychological effects of bullying and sexual harassment. Specifically, her academic progress was negatively affected by being subjected to sexual harassment and she started experiencing depression. Phoebe's family should help her seek counseling for mental health concerns around depressed mood and self-harming behaviors. Treatment will likely help Phoebe understand how her thoughts and emotions are triggering negative coping strategies such as cutting her arms and legs.

For the academic impact, Phoebe's family might need to explore whether it is safe for her to remain at school. The student in Minnesota continued to experience harassment in high school in retaliation for fighting her case. Therefore, Phoebe might benefit from being removed from the situation entirely by moving schools or being in a home school arrangement.

2. RICHARD IS BULLIED ON SOCIAL MEDIA

Richard who is in high school in Alabama finds that he is a fish out of water when it comes to his classmates. The other boys go out of their way to show their masculinity and act in stereotypical ways to prove their heterosexuality. They intentionally and openly brag about sexual exploits and describe their female classmates in great sexual detail. In fact, their ability to "bed" girls in high school has become a competition of sorts. Those high school boys not willing to play along are easily exposed and have become targets of teasing and threats.

Not only was Richard not raised to talk about the intimate details of close relationships, but he also fears being outed by his peers. Richard has kept his sexual identity as a gay male secret as he knows he would face name-calling and be subjected to incessant bullying and possibly even violent attacks. In school, he notices that his peers incorporate homophobic language in their everyday conversation. They will use words like "fag" or say "that's so gay" without a second thought. Lately some of his peers have begun to suspect that Richard is gay. They have called him out in pretty obvious ways by trying to coax him into making sexist comments about female classmates. They ask him which females should be placed on the "top 10 females who are most f%@$able" list, and when he does not respond, they ask him, "What? Are you gay or something? That's disgusting and not natural, Richard."

Richard has observed firsthand that sexual harassment can be not only a way to keep girls and women in their place but also a way to reinforce masculinity and the importance of being straight. Because he refuses to participate in the derogatory remarks about his female peers, he discovers that people are posting comments on social media platforms calling him out and labeling him as queer. Richard is becoming increasingly more frustrated and fearful of his identity being revealed publicly. His parents are strictly conservative and will not approve of his sexual identity. It is literally not safe to come out of the closet. Richard is developing severe anxiety and starting to develop fantasies of taking his life so he can escape the discomfort. What should Richard do?

Analysis

A straightforward interpretation of this case is that Richard is the victim of cyber bullying. Like in other forms of bullying, there are often severe mental health consequences. Unlike bullying that happened prior to the internet and the strong social media presence, cyber bullying can take place at any hour of the day. In other words, Richard is never safe from the words and posts of his peers. To make matters worse, Richard is experiencing homophobic slurs and feeling "outed" by his bullies.

It is recommended that Richard finds a safe person to talk to about what he is experiencing. He can call a teen suicide hotline to get immediate help. Connecting with an online LBGTQIA group will provide validation and additional resources. There are some support groups offered on social media that might be a way to connect with others experiencing similar kinds of bullying while remaining anonymous. It is advised that Richard finds an avenue to receive professional counseling to deal with his severe anxiety and to assess whether he should be hospitalized for his protection.

Richard will probably want to discontinue his social media accounts or unfriend the offenders. However, working with a counselor to develop coping strategies and to understand the avenues available to report abuse when it has occurred would also help. Each school is now required to have a Title IX coordinator for reporting sexual harassment and bullying. Moreover, teachers and school counselors are obligated to report situations if they become aware of them.

Although helping victims with mental health concerns is important for dealing with bullying and sexual harassment, it is only part of the recommended solution. It is a school's obligation to foster a safe learning environment. Schools who are serious about maintaining the safety of students and bullying prevention should take several intentional steps.

1.   Schools must develop policies around discrimination of LBGTQ students. Not only should harassment be prohibited, but there also must be a clear procedure for reporting incidents when they occur.
2.   Schools must create an inclusive environment for LBGTQ students. Teachers and staff must be trained on how to recognize bullying, discrimination, and harassment.
3.   Schools must show open support for LBGTQ and take a stand against discrimination in visible ways. Examples include having a designated day, creating safe zones (that are visibly marked with stickers or signage), or developing LBGTQ-inclusive curricula.
4.   Schools can support the development of ally groups and student organizations for LBGTQ students. These groups can help validate shared experiences and help LBGTQ students to feel less isolated and alone.

These steps would be helpful for Richard to navigate his feelings around sexual identity and to create a safe space at school that is free of bullying and sexual harassment.

3. ALICIA HAS A CREEPY BOSS

Alicia is a 15-year-old high school student in a mid-sized city in South-eastern North Carolina. She self-identifies as biracial with a Caucasian mother and Black father. Alicia recognizes that her skin tone is a light chocolate color that resembles a golden tan and that she has light-colored eyes. People have told her since childhood that she looks exotic, which has led to mixed feelings. On the one hand, she feels special and appreciates being unique. However, on the other hand, she often feels like she does not fit in with any one group or belong anywhere. Sometimes her Black friends will tell her she acts "too white" when she shares her music preferences. She has noticed that some of the Caucasian boys in her class treat her differently than her white classmates as if she is somehow inferior due to her skin color. She also has been called a fair number of names like "honey bear," "chocolate bear," and "Hershey's kiss."

Alicia is used to being evaluated for her appearance and has become numb to many of the comments that come her way. To earn money toward college, she decides to apply for a job at the Publix grocery store near her house for some after-school employment. In the interview, the store manager is surprised when Alicia correctly identifies fennel and shallots and is able to distinguish between different kinds of herbs. "I wouldn't have thought you would know that," he ventures. She guesses her future boss is simply thinking that at her young age she would not be as wise around the kitchen, but Alicia has been preparing extravagant recipes from a young age.

On her first day of work, Alicia puts on her uniform with giddy anticipation. Her polyester shirt is formfitting and shows the contours of her breasts, but she can tuck in the shirt with no problem. When Alicia comes into work, one of the female employees asks her who hired her. When Alicia provides the name of the male store manager, the coworker responds knowingly, "It figures." Alicia feels a little discouraged as she knows that she earned the job on her own merit as well as her knowledge of items in the produce department.

Toward the end of her first week on the job, the store manager who hired her comes up to the cash register behind her. He breathes on her neck and asks how things are going for her at the new job. Then he proceeds to hover around longer than what would be natural or comfortable. His hand briefly grazes her arm and he moves on. She bristles at his touch but figures he probably did not mean anything by it. Alicia reasons that if anything he is a father-like figure nearly 20 years her senior. He is probably just being supportive, Alicia figures.

Several weeks later, Alicia finds herself in the break room alone with the store manager. He smiles widely and winks at her before saying, "If you are nice to me, I'll give you the best schedule." She laughs in a strained sort of way and quickly exits the room. Alicia remains on the floor for the duration of her shift. She finds that she is conflicted about whether to resign from the job, play along with the store manager's antics, or try to avoid him entirely. This is a difficult decision for her as if she quits her cashier job she would need to forgo earnings for her college savings account, and it is too late in the summer to get another job. It also means that having her store manager as a reference would be challenging if she leaves her employment without notice. What should she do?

Analysis

Like other individuals who have experienced sexual harassment at work, Alicia likely feels powerless, and it is natural to feel conflicted about the best way to respond. Regardless of what next steps she takes, Alicia is likely going to have to deal with feeling some degree of shame or guilt that she somehow brought this upon herself. However, it is important that Alicia recognizes that the behaviors of her store manager meet the very definition of what constitutes sexual harassment in the workplace. Therefore, several recommendations should be taken into consideration.

1. Alicia should document the incidents very carefully with as much detail as possible. If she is aware of witnesses to situations she has experienced or the possibility that someone overheard her exchanges with her manager, she should note that as well.
2. As difficult as it is, Alicia should make every effort to make it clear that these sexual advances are unwelcome. Whether it is special attention or being asked out for a date, Alicia should make it be known that the answer is an emphatic "no."
3. If she is not already aware of her company's policy and procedure for reporting sexual harassment, Alicia should research how one would go about submitting a complaint against her manager. This information is likely available in an employee handbook or the onboarding materials. Usually how to report is outlined and involves making a complaint to a supervisor's supervisor, to the human resources department, or using an employee hotline.
4. It might be suggested for Alicia to seek legal consultation from a firm that specializes in workplace concerns. This independent route

is especially recommended if the organization has been known to hide previous complaints or perpetuates a culture of sexual harassment and power inequities.

5.   Alicia should find a support network to help with emotions associated with sexual harassment and working in a threatening climate. These supportive others should provide a safe space for Alicia to weigh her options for the next way forward and to discuss the sexual harassment she has endured.

6.   It may be helpful for Alicia to seek professional help to deal with anger, frustration, and guilt she may be experiencing associated with the incidents she has encountered at work. It is not uncommon for victims of sexual harassment to experience intense anxiety, depression, and some level of trauma. A healthy step is talking through her experiences so that she can start the journey of moving on.

4. LAUREN IS TARGETED BECAUSE OF HER CURVES

Lauren has always been curvaceous for as long as she can remember. Adults and kids tend to overestimate her age because of her bodily appearance and maturing earlier than her peers. As a seventh grader, Lauren notices that many of the girls in her class bring different outfits to school and change when they arrive. These girls also apply makeup once they get to school and scrub it off before they go home for the day. Lauren is fortunate that she enjoys open communications with her mother, who is permissive about wearing tasteful amounts of makeup and shopping for clothing that is on trend.

In fact, Lauren's mother takes her shopping before the first day of school for a mother-daughter day. They get makeovers and have pedicures at a local spa. Her mother takes her to a local department store, and they try on numerous outfits. Her mother encourages her to buy a variety of skirts, blouses, and pants. All abide by the specified dress code for the junior high school Lauren will be attending. The first day of school Lauren selects one of her new outfits, which is a brightly colored mini skirt and matching top. It fits her perfectly and shows off her small waist but hugs her hips in the right places. When Lauren walks into school, she feels all eyes turn to her. Feeling proud, she stands a little taller as she approaches her locker. Soon the gazes from her classmates turn to cat calls. As she walks into homeroom, she is disgusted when one of her male classmates says, "Hey girl—wanna sit on my lap?"

Later in the day, she is called to the principal's office. She figures word has gotten back about the poor behavior of her peers and prepares to report the specifics. Instead Principal Johnson leads in, "We are going to need you to go home and change your clothes to something more appropriate for school." When Lauren asks which dress code she is violating with her outfit, Mr. Johnson is at a loss on how to respond and clearly seems uncomfortable. "You look very adult," he admits. And then he asks, "Do your parents know what you have on today?" When Lauren explains her shopping trip and that her mother picked out the outfit, Mr. Johnson continues to remain steadfast that the outfit is not suitable for the school setting. Lauren, feeling humiliated, goes home and changes into something else. She never wears her skirt set to school again.

It is unsurprising that Lauren's curvy figure has been receiving attention from boys for the past couple of years. At first, she was excited about being able to buy a training bra and relished the opportunity to have a special shopping day with her mother. They traveled to Victoria's Secret so that Lauren could get measured for her bra size and to pick out garments that fit her personal style and in fun colors. Unfortunately, her excitement waned when the same boys began to tease her mercilessly by saying, "I can see your bra!" When she is least expecting it, these boys, or other boys from her grade, come up to her and snap her bra strap. Not only does it sting when the band cuts back into her skin but also Lauren experiences shame and grows red with embarrassment. She tells her mother about the incident as well as the taunting she experienced on the first day of school.

Her mother sets up an appointment with Mr. Johnson to discuss the bullying by her classmates. To Lauren's chagrin, the principal's response to Lauren's mother is "Boys will be boys. This is the age when they begin to notice the fairer sex. Wouldn't you agree?" Even worse is his serious recommendation for Lauren to avoid dressing like she was trying to get their attention. "It is like you are wearing a flag to wave them down and get them to notice you."

In an attempt to hide her body from lewd comments and peering eyeballs down the front, Lauren begins to wear baggy shirts that do not show the form of her breasts. Lauren has always been hypersensitive to comments about her body, but now she feels intense dissatisfaction about her body parts that feature feminine characteristics. She looks at herself in the mirror with disgust. She makes sure not to wear anything too revealing, formfitting, or low cut because she does not want to give the wrong idea or appear to be seeking the attention of others. Her confidence drops and she feels self-conscious. She has learned quickly that women are blamed for bringing on negative attention from their male counterparts. What should she do?

Analysis

Lauren's case unfortunately represents a common tendency for others to blame the victims of sexual harassment. Clearly, Lauren is the recipient of verbal bullying and comments as well as physical bullying and unwanted sexual attention (e.g., snapping of bra strap). Rather than being supported by an adult authority figure, Lauren is treated as the person to be blamed and is encouraged to change her clothes. This example depicts how schools can contribute to the problem and participate in a vicious cycle when it comes to discrimination against girls and women. Lauren learns from these incidents that it is her duty to hide her body under baggy clothing and, worse, that she should be ashamed of her curves and womanly features. These messages become internalized, have a devastating impact on her self-confidence, and put Lauren at risk for all kinds of mental health concerns. Lauren will likely be more vulnerable to developing body image disturbances, disordered eating behaviors, self-harming behaviors such as cutting, and substance use disorders. She may ultimately meet the clinical diagnosis of mental disorders such as mood disorders and anxiety disorders. Adolescents are at an increased risk for suicidal thinking and tendencies.

Given how fragile Lauren is, it is important that she have a strong support network. Lauren's mother should help her find a licensed professional counselor who specializes in treating teenagers and has expertise in eating disorders and body image concerns. She should be assessed for body image concerns and eating behaviors as well as other unhealthy coping strategies. The counselor can help confront negative thoughts that Lauren is likely to direct at herself in response to these incidents with her peers and the school administrator. Lauren will need to address shame and guilt associated with sexual harassment.

Lauren and her mother can also take some additional steps to address sexual harassment in school. The following areas are recommended:

1. Lauren should document the behaviors she has witnessed and personally experienced at school. She should include notes on her actions and responses to reporting the incidents to the principal. She can record any emails or correspondence.
2. If she experiences further sexual harassment, she should continue to clearly state "no" and express that she feels uncomfortable.

3.   File a complaint with the Department of Education. If there is a Title IX coordinator, that person should be notified immediately. If there is a trusted teacher or school counselor, Lauren can report the situation to them.
4.   It is recommended that Lauren's family seek legal consultation for the case so that an independent perspective is provided.
5.   Lauren is likely to face an uphill battle while she reports the sexual harassment and must prepare for an intense line of questioning. There may be negative responses from some of her classmates. She needs to have plenty of support for whatever daggers come her way. This will not be an easy road for Lauren, but it is important that she receive the message from family, friends, and important others that she is not to blame.

5. JAMIE IS HARASSED ON THE TENNIS TEAM

Jamie, who is 17 years old, has made the college tennis team. She is excited about the transition from high school to college, and to move out of her home state of Maryland to a small town in South Carolina. She had met her roommate at the Honors College event and stayed in contact prior to the move. They had coordinated about the colors for bed comforters and dormitory furniture. Now that she has arrived at campus, Jamie feels overwhelmed. Her tennis team has lots of practices, which is fine, but there are also social activities. The coach encourages the team to eat together and to do activities outside of practice like yoga classes and movie nights. She finds it exhausting to spend so much time with her teammates, and it does not allow her much time for anything else. Her homework is slipping and given that she wants to complete the honor's program, her classes are more challenging than many of her teammates' classes. She has already taken the necessary Advanced Placement exams to waive some of the general classes.

Jamie feels so stressed about academics as well as being away from her family. Her coach, Josh, who is in his twenties has been the "big brother away from home." Josh is always willing to stay after practice to talk to her about her hard classes and worries about flunking out of school. He tells her that he has a younger sister and wants to look after her since she is so far from home. This is reassuring to Jamie, who often feels alone and isolated. She also secretly enjoys the attention from an older guy who is considered the "cool coach" by her teammates. She has overheard the other tennis players talking about Josh in graphic and sexually explicit ways.

Jamie never participates in their conversations but feels a little superior to her teammates for the unique relationship she shares with the coach.

Initially Jamie and Josh just sit on the bleachers and talk about topics. Then on one night after practice Josh goes back to his truck and pulls out a six pack. He hands her a can of beer even though she is underaged. When she shares that she is having trouble staying awake to do her homework, he shares caffeine pills with her. He buys her and her roommate a bottle of champagne when she reveals it is her birthday weekend. Despite their friendship, nothing physical begins for over six months. Eventually Josh offers her a hug when she is feeling particularly down. This turns into a pat on the head, a kiss on the cheek, a shoulder massage. They have started spending more time together on the weekends. Josh drives her out to the lake for fishing or boating. They grab a bite to eat at the local Steak and Waffle restaurant.

Jamie has never had a serious boyfriend and craves companionship. When Josh begins to repeatedly ask her out, Jamie begins to feel uncomfortable. He implies that she owes him a date or sexual favors for the special attention he has given her. He grows frustrated when she expresses viewing him as a friend or brother. His negative emotions rise, and the more she resists his advances, he threatens to take away her scholarship or put other players in the doubles' tournament. Gone is the friendly demeanor and the supportive older brother persona. Josh is treating her differently in practices and the other players are acting openly hostile. They assume that she and Josh are sleeping together. What should Jamie do?

Analysis

It is normal for a new college student to experience stress and loneliness during their transition from high school to the college environment. In Jamie's case, she has moved to a new state and has newfound freedom away from her family. After being successful in high school sports and academics, she is in an entirely new place. She shows evidence of being a high achiever in her desire to pursue the honor's program while maintaining her status as a student athlete on a college campus. Unfortunately, with these transitions, Jamie has become vulnerable and an easy target for predators like her coach, Josh. Josh recognizes that Jamie does not have immediate family or friends to "call out" this unusual relationship with her coach. He also knows from experience that women have been socialized to receive certain validation from the attention of men, especially those in a power position. It is likely that Jamie is not the first victim of her tennis coach.

Josh's stance of acting like a supportive "big brother" is classic predator behavior. He is approachable, youthful, and shows an interest in Jamie. To Jamie, who is naive and trying to adapt to a new environment and culture, his attentions are interpreted as being a caring mentor. Jamie knows that it is not uncommon for athletes to have a close relationship with their coaches. A red flag, however, should be the amount of alone time she is spending with the coach as well as his supply of alcoholic beverages. Josh is clearly grooming Jamie to develop a sexual relationship over time. Like other predators, he is patient and works to gain the trust of his victim who should have every right to believe in her college coach.

When a coach asks out a player, it is inappropriate. The coach is in a position of power and has control over playing time, whether the experience on the team is positive or negative, and at the extreme may influence whether students can keep their scholarship. This means in simple language that a coach should not be asking out a player. Jamie will likely grapple with an internal struggle associated with appreciating and valuing the attention she received while feeling guilty for not reciprocating his sexual advances. She will likely wonder if she led on her coach or gave him a signal that she was interested in him "that way."

To help Jamie cope with the various feelings she will experience, it is recommended that she seek counseling. As a college student, she will have access to a university counseling center. The treatment professionals who work there will be obligated to maintain confidentiality of her sessions, but she may find solace in a referral outside of the university. This separation may help her to feel more comfortable sharing the experiences in a relatively small community. She can work with that individual to explore resources available to report what has happened to her.

In addition to receiving counseling, Jamie should be encouraged to practice all forms of self-care including developing a consistent sleeping schedule and eliminating the use of caffeine pills so that her body can achieve a more natural rhythm. This may mean that she will need to adjust her schedule to identify blocks to devote time to study sessions. It may be recommended that Jamie develop some friendships outside of tennis so that she has a stronger support system. She will need to explore whether it is in her best personal interest to remain on the tennis team and to stay at her current university. She will be encouraged to identify some healthy coping skills and strategies to replace the unhealthy relationship with her coach.

Glossary

Ableism: Represents discrimination against individuals with disabilities.

Arbitration: A form of resolution for disputes that involves having a neutral party make a decision regarding the merits of the case in question.

Civil Rights Act in 1964: Refers to the United States making sexual harassment illegal and considered to be a form of gender discrimination.

Contrapower Harassment: When a subordinate in a lower-status role harasses their superior or someone in a higher-status role. An example of this would be a student who harasses their teacher or counselor in school.

The Dark Triad: Refers to psychological characteristics of narcissism, psychopathy, and Machiavellianism.

Defamation: Refers to an oral (i.e., slander) or written false statement about a person's character with intent to damage their reputation.

Equal Employment Opportunity Commission (EEOC): A federal agency in the United States whose work is to administer and enforce laws for gender identity and sexual orientation as other protected classes (e.g., sex, age, race, national origin, religion, disability) in the workplace.

Heterosexism: Refers to discriminatory acts against individuals due to their sexual orientation or gender identity.

Homophobic Slurs: A negative comment about one's sexual orientation.

Hostile Environment: When the presence of sexual harassment makes one's work environment toxic or intolerable.

LBGTQIA: Refers to individuals who self-identify as LBGTQ (stands for Lesbian Bisexual Gay Trans Queer Intersex Ally).

Machiavellianism: Refers to being deceptive and acting without morals.

Mandatory Arbitration Clause: Contract that is signed with one's employer in which employee waives their right to litigation (i.e., jury trial) for a sexual harassment claim. This clause is a controversial way to reach resolution that is thought to benefit the employer more than the employee.

Mediation: A form of third-party neutral intervention that involves having parties in conflict to meet to explore options and discuss the issues with the goal of reaching a resolution.

#MeToo: A movement that brought public attention to sexual harassment and assault.

Moral Disengagement: Refers to a perpetrator characteristic where rules do not apply to the harasser because they have created her own version of reality that includes a separate set of rules that inevitably justify one's behavior.

Narcissistic: Refers to a perpetrator who is overly consumed within themselves, displays a lack of empathy, and cannot understand the views of others.

Posttraumatic Stress Disorder (PTSD): A psychological disorder associated with a history of trauma or traumatic event.

Psychopathy: Defined as a behavior or trait associated with being manipulative, aggressive, and impulsive.

Quid Pro Quo Sexual Harassment: Refers to the expectation of sexual favors in exchange for professional advantage (e.g., job promotion).

RAINN (Rape, Abuse & Incest National Network): Refers to an organization that provides a myriad of resources to learn more about what a person might expect if they have faced sexual harassment, for providing support to survivors of sexual harassment.

Retaliation: When an employee receives negative treatment or is disadvantaged in some way within the work setting after making a complaint about their supervisor, another colleague, or their employer.

Sexual Favoritism: For this form of sexual harassment, the employer only rewards employees who submit to sexual demands. Other employees who refuse are denied promotion or raises.

Sexually Explicit Talk: Refers to someone regardless of gender making sexual innuendos (e.g., references to sex in the course of a conversation).

STIs (Sexually Transmitted Diseases): Refers to specific sexually diseases, such as human papillomavirus HPV (i.e., genital warts), chlamydia, and HSV-2 genital herpes.

Title IX of the Educational Amendments of 1972: Refers to the law that attempts to prevent any discrimination on the basis of sex and protects both male and female students. This law has been often associated with gender equality in sports.

Title VII of the Civil Rights Act of 1964: Refers to the part of the law that covers an employment context that was initially for targeting discrimination that women faced in the workplace; however, it covers both gender discrimination of women and men.

Totality-of-Circumstances Test: An assessment used to determine whether the conduct results in hostile environment. This test includes the evaluation of the following factors: 1) frequency of discriminatory conduct; 2) severity; 3) whether the behavior is humiliating or physically threatening; and 4) whether the sexual harassing behavior creates disruption or interference with the work performance of the victim.

Umbrella Term: Refers to a wide spectrum of behaviors ranging from requests for sexual favors within the workplace in exchange for promotion opportunities to teasing a person about their appearance to groping.

Whistleblowing: The disclosure of questionable practices that may meet the definition of illegal, immoral, or illegitimate by current or former employees.

White Privilege: Refers to a term that has been used to characterize the subtle and obvious ways that life experiences may be different for people based on the color of one's skin.

Workplace Romance: Romantic relationship that starts or occurs in the workplace.

Directory of Resources

BOOKS

Be Fierce: Stop Harassment and Take Your Power Back
Author: Gretchen Carlson
Publisher: Center Street; Year: 2017
ISBN: 1478992158 ISBN-13: 9781478992158
Website: https://www.centerstreet.com/

Sexual Harassment: A Reference Handbook
Author: Merril D. Smith
Publisher: ABC-CLIO; Year: 2020
ISBN: 1440867704 ISBN-13: 9781440867705
Website: https://products.abc-clio.com/

Sexual Harassment in Education and Work Settings: Current Research and Best Practices for Prevention
Author: Michele A. Paludi, Jennifer L. Martin, James E. Gruber, and Susan Fineran
Publisher: ABC-CLIO; Year: 2015
ISBN: 1440832943 ISBN-13: 9781440832949
Website: https://products.abc-clio.com/

She Said: Breaking the Sexual Harassment Story That Helped Ignite a Movement

Author: Jodi Kantor and Megan Twohey
Publisher: Penguin Press; Year: 2019
ISBN: 0525560343 ISBN-13: 9780525560340
Website: https://www.penguinrandomhouse.com/books/

Stop Telling Women to Smile: Stories of Street Harassment and How We're Taking Back Our Power

Author: Tatyana Fazlalizadeh
Publisher: Basics Books; Year: 2020
ISBN: 1580058485 ISBN-13: 9781580058483
Website: https://www.basicbooks.com/

*You Too?: 25 Voices Share Their #MeToo Stories

Author: Janet Gurtler
Publisher: Inkyard Press; Year: 2020
ISBN: 1335929088 ISBN-13: 9781335929082
Website: https://www.harlequin.com/

JOURNALS

Gender & Society

Publisher: Sage
Website: https://journals.sagepub.com/home/gas

Journal of Clinical Sport Psychology

Special issue: Sexual harassment and assault in sport (June 2019, Volume 13, Issue 2)
Publisher: Human Kinetics
Website: https://journals.humankinetics.com/view/journals/jcsp/13/2/jcsp.13.issue-2.xml

Violence Against Women (VAW)

Publisher: Sage
Website: https://journals.sagepub.com/home/vawa

HELPLINES/HOTLINES

*Childhelp National Child Abuse Hotline

Phone/Text: 1-800-4-A-CHILD or 1-800-422-4453
Website: https://www.childhelp.org/hotline/
A resource if you are being hurt, know someone who might be hurting, or are afraid you might hurt another.

LGBT National Help Center

Phone: 1-888-843-4564 (LGBT National Hotline)
1-800-246-7743 (LGBT National Youth Hotline)
1-88-234-7243 (LGBT National Senior Hotline)
Website: http://glnh.org/
Serving the lesbian, gay, bisexual, transgender, queer, and questioning community by providing free and confidential peer support and local resources.

National Domestic Violence Hotline

Phone: 1-800-799-SAFE (7233) TTY: 1-800-787-3224
Website: https://www.thehotline.org/ Text: "LOVEIS" to 22522
Offers support for people living in violent situations and referrals for additional services. Available in Spanish.

National Drug and Alcohol Abuse Hotline

Phone: 1-877-882-9275
Website: https://www.drug-rehabs.org/
A referral and resource if you or a loved one are struggling with drug addiction or alcoholism.

National Human Trafficking Resource Center Hotline

Phone: 1-888-373-7888
Website: https://humantraffickinghotline.org/
Hotline for a victim of human trafficking.

*National Runaway Safeline

Phone: 1-800-RUNAWAY (786-2929)
Website: https://www.1800runaway.org/#
Hotline with resources for youth, teens, parents, and guardians.

National Suicide Prevention Lifeline

Phone: 1-800-273-8255
Website: http://suicidepreventionlifeline.org/
Provides 24/7 free and confidential support for people in distress, prevention and crisis resources for you and your loved ones, and best practices for professionals.

Rape, Abuse, & Incest National Network (RAINN)

1220 L Street, NW Suite 505, Washington, DC 20005 USA
Phone: 1-800-656-HOPE (4673) Chat: https://hotline.rainn.org/online
Website: www.rainn.org En Español: https://www.rainn.org/es
Nation's largest anti-sexual violence organization, resources, and hotline.

Safe Helpline for Department of Defense (DOD) Community

Attention: DoD Safe Helpline
1220 L Street, NW Suite 505, Washington, DC 20005 USA
Phone: 1-877-995-5247 Chat: https://safehelpline.org/live-chat
Website: https://safehelpline.org/ Safe Helpline App: Apple Store/Google Play
Hotline, support, information, resources, self-care exercises for members of the DoD community affected by sexual assault.

Stronghearts Native Helpline

Phone: 1-844-762-8483
Website: https://www.strongheartshelpline.org/
Advocacy for culturally appropriate, free, and confidential service for Native Americans affected by domestic violence and dating violence.

*TEEN LINE

Phone: 1-310-855-HOPE (4673) or 1-800-TLC-TEEN (852-8336)
Text: "TEEN" to 839863 TEEN TALK APP: free on iPhone
Website: https://teenlineonline.org/
A nonprofit, community-based organization helping troubled teenagers address their problems.

Trans Lifeline

Phone: 1-877-565-8860 Canada: 1-877-330-6366
Website: https://www.translifeline.org/
The Trans Lifeline is dedicated to the well-being of transgender people.

*Trevor Project (LBGT Youth Crisis Line)

Phone: 1-866-488-7386 Text: "START" to 678678
Website: https://www.thetrevorproject.org/
A young LGBTQ support hotline for suicide and support.

VictimConnect Resource Center

Phone: 1-855-4-VICTIM (1-855-484-2846)
Website: https://victimconnect.org/ Online chat: Chat.VictimConnect.org
A referral helpline where crime victims can learn about their rights and options confidentially and compassionately. A program of the National Center for Victims of Crime.

ORGANIZATIONS

American Arbitration Association

Phone: 1-800-778-7879
Website: https://www.adr.org/
Not-for-profit private global provider of alternative dispute resolution services in the world.

American Association of University Women

1310 L St. NW, Suite 1000 Washington, DC 20005
Phone: 1-202-785-7700
Website: https://www.aauw.org/
An organization since 1881 advocating for women and girls for fair pay and economic opportunity for women to end discrimination.

American Bar Association (ABA)

Phone: 1-800-285-2221 International: +1-312-988-5000
Email: Service@americanbar.org Website: https://www.americanbar.org/
Serving equally their members, their profession, and the public by defending liberty and delivering justice as the national representative of the legal profession.

American Civil Liberties Union (ACLU)

125 Broad Street, 18th Floor New York, NY 10004
Phone: 1-212-549-2500
Website: https://www.aclu.org/
An organization dedicated to the preservation and protection of individual civil liberties and civil rights.

American Federation of Labor and Congress of Industrial Organizations (AFL-CIO America's Union)

815 16ᵗʰ St. NW Washington, DC 20006
Text: "WORK" to 235246
Website: https://aflcio.org/
Nonprofit organization to ensure all working people are treated fairly, with decent paychecks and benefits, safe jobs, dignity, and equal opportunities.

American Psychiatric Association (APA)

Phone: 1-888-35-PSYCH or 1-888-357-7924
Outside the U.S. and Canada: 703-907-7300 Website: www.psych.org
Organization of psychiatrists working together to ensure humane care and effective treatment for all persons with mental illness, including substance use disorders.

American Psychology Association (APA)

750 First St. NE Washington, DC 20002-4242 USA
Phone: 1-800-374-2721 or 202-336-5500 TDD/TTY: 202-336-6123
Website: www.apa.org
Scientific and professional organization representing psychology in the United States.

Anderson-Davis, Inc.

Phone: 1-310-451-0636 Email: info@andersondavis.com
Website: https://www.andersondavis.com/
An educational services and consulting firm specializing in areas of sexual harassment.

Asian-American Legal Defense and Education Fund (AALDEF)

99 Hudson St, 12ᵗʰ Floor New York, NY 10013
Phone: 1-212-966-5932 Email: https://www.aaldef.org/
Website: https://www.aaldef.org/
A national organization founded in 1974, protects and promotes the civil rights of Asian Americans including sexual harassment and discrimination.

Association for Talent Development (ATD)

Phone: 1-800-628-2783 International: 1-703-683-8100
Email: customercar@td.org Website: https://www.td.org/
A national organization of professional workplace trainers and resources on sexual harassment training.

Centers for Disease Control and Prevention (CDC: Sexual Violence)

1600 Clifton Road Atlanta, GA 30333 USA
Phone: 800-CDC-INFO (800-232-4636) TTY: (888) 232-6348
Email: https://wwwn.cdc.gov/dcs/contactus/form
Website: https://www.cdc.gov/violenceprevention/sexualviolence/
Information on sexual harassment.

Equal Rights Advocates

1170 Market St., Suite 700, San Francisco CA 94102
Phone: 1-415-471-1472 Email: advice@equalrights.org
Website: https://www.equalrights.org/ Online: Referral form
Organization that advocates for gender justice in workplaces and schools
across the country.

Feminist Majority Foundation (FMJ)

1600 Wilson Boulevard, Suite 101, Arlington, VA 22209 USA
Phone: 1-703-522-2214
Website: https://www.feminist.org/
Organization dedicated to women's equality, reproductive health, nonvi-
olence, and resources.

Institute for Women's Policy Research (IWPR)

1200 19th Street NW, Suite 301 Washington, DC 20036
Phone: 1-202-785-5100 Email: iwpr@iwpr.org
Website: https://iwpr.org/
An organization conducting research to inspire public dialogue,
shape policy, and improve the lives and opportunities of women of
diverse backgrounds, circumstances, and experiences including sexual
harassment.

Making Caring Common (MCC), Harvard Graduate School of Education

14 Appian Way, Cambridge, MA 02138 USA
Phone: 1-617-284-9544 Email: mcc@gse.harvard.edu
Website: https://mcc.gse.harvard.edu/
A project to create a more caring world; come to understand and seek
fairness and justice with tips, resources lists, discussion guides, and more;
use with kids and others.

Mexican American Legal Defense and Educational Fund (MALDEF)

Headquarters in Los Angeles, CA with regional offices throughout United States
Phone: 1-213-629-2512 Email: info@MALDEF.org
Website: https://www.maldef.org/
Nation's leading Latino legal civil rights organization.

NAACP Legal Defense and Educational Fund, Inc. (LDF)

40 Rector Street, 5th Floor New York, NY 10006
Phone: 1-212-965-2000
Website: https://www.naacpldf.org/
An organization fighting for racial justice as well as referrals for sexual harassment claims.

National Adult Protective Services Association (NAPSA)

Website: http://www.napsa-now.org/
Formed in 1989, the goal of NAPSA is to provide Adult Protective Services (APS) programs a forum for sharing information, solving problems, and improving the quality of services for victims of elder and vulnerable adult mistreatment.

National Bar Association

1816 12th Street NW, Washington D.C. 20009 USA
Phone: 1-202-842-3900
Website: https://nationalbar.org/
Nation's oldest and largest network of predominantly African American attorneys and judges.

National Center for Victims of Crime

P.O. Box 101207, Arlington, VA 22210 USA
Phone: 1-202-467-8700 Email: info@victimsofcrime.org
Website: https://victimsofcrime.org/
Nonprofit organization that advocates for victims' rights, trains professionals who work with victims, and serves as a trusted source of information on victims' issues.

National Coalition Against Domestic Violence (NCADV)

600 Grant, Suite 750, Denver, CO 80203
Phone: 1-303-839-1852
Website: http://www.ncadv.org/

An organization to lead, mobilize, and raise our voices to support efforts that demand a change of conditions that lead to domestic violence such as patriarchy, privilege, racism, sexism, and classism.

National Immigration Project for the National Lawyers Guild
Website: https://nipnlg.org/
Organization that provides legal and technical support to immigrant communities, legal practitioners, and all advocates seeking to advance the rights of noncitizens.

National Institute of Mental Health (NIMH)
Science Writing, Press, and Dissemination Branch
6001 Executive Blvd., Room 6200, MSC 9663 Bethesda, MD 20892-9663 USA
Phone: 1-866-615-6464 TTY: 1-866-415-8051 Fax: 301-443-4279
Email: nimhinfo@nih.gov Website: https://www.nimh.nih.gov/index.shtml
Information for the understanding and treatment of mental illness.

National Institutes of Health (NIH)
9000 Rockville Pike Bethesda, MD 20892 USA Website: https://www.nih.gov/
Nation's medical research agency, supporting scientific studies that turn discovery into health.

National Organization for Men Against Sexism
Website: https://nomas.org/
An organization of men and women supporting positive changes for men by advocating a perspective that is pro-feminist, gay affirmative, anti-racist, dedicated to enhancing men's lives and committed to justice on a broad range of social issues including class, age, religion, and physical abilities.

National Sexual Violence Resource Center (NSVRC)
2101 N. Front Street Governor's Plaza North, Building #2, Harrisburg, PA 17110 USA
Phone: 717-909-0710 or 1-877-739-3895 TTY: 717-909-0715 Fax: 717-909-0714
Website: http://www.nsvrc.org/
Advocates and sex offender treatment professionals' network.

National Women's Law Center

11 Dupont Circle NW, Suite 800, Washington, DC 20036
Phone: 1-202-588-5180 Seeking Legal Help: 1-202-319-3053
Website: https://nwlc.org/
Organization of advocates, experts, and lawyers who fight for gender justice, especially for women facing multiple forms of discrimination.

9 to 5: National Association of Working Woman

Phone: 1-800-522-0925 Email: helpline@9to5.org
Website: https://9to5.org/
National membership organizations of working women in the United States, dedicated to putting working women's issues on the public agenda.

Protect Our Defenders

950 N. Washington Street, Alexandria, VA 22314
Email: info@protectourdefenders.org
Website: https://www.protectourdefenders.com/
The only national organization solely dedicated to ending the epidemic of rape and sexual assault in the military and to combating a culture to pervasive misogyny, sexual harassment, and retribution against victims.

U.S. Department of Labor Women's Bureau

200 Constitution Avenue NW, Room S-3002, Washington, DC 20210 USA
Phone: 1-800-827-5335
Website: https://www.dol.gov/agencies/wb Email: womens.bureau@dol.gov
An agency that develops policies and standards and conducts inquiries to safeguard the interests of working women; to advocate for their equality and economic security for themselves and their families; and to promote quality work environments.

U.S. Equal Employment Opportunity Commission (EEOC)

131 M Street NE, Washington, DC 20507 USA
Phone: 1-800-669-4000 TTY: 1-800-669-6820 ASL: 1-844-234-5122
Website: https://www.eeoc.gov/ Email: info@eeoc.gov
Responsible for enforcing all federal laws that apply to all types of work situations, including hiring, firing, promotions, harassment, training, wages, and benefits.

World Health Organization (WHO)

Website: http://www.who.int/topics/en/ Twitter: https://twitter.com/who
Facebook: https://www.facebook.com/WHO
Organization and resources about projects, initiatives, activities on health
and development topics.

WEBSITES

*About-Face

P.O. Box 191145 San Francisco, CA 94102 USA
Phone: 415-448-6263 Website: www.about-face.org
Tools to understand and resist harmful media messages that affect self-esteem.

*Advocates for Youth

Website: https://advocatesforyouth.org/
Online resource for youth and educators to make informed and responsible decisions about their reproductive, sexual health, and family life education program.

Battered Women's Justice Project

Website: https://www.bwjp.org/
A project that offers training, technical assistance, and consultation on the most promising practices of the criminal and civil justice systems in addressing domestic violence.

Befrienders Worldwide

Website: https://www.befrienders.org/ Email: info@befrienders.org
Online worldwide referral resource for individuals in distress needing support via helplines, SMS messages, face-to-face, internet, chat, outreach, and local partnerships

Better Man Conference

Website: https://bettermanconference.com/
An event with resources, support, and community to engage men as allies in creating an inclusive culture.

*Break the Cycle

Website: http://www.breakthecycle.org/
Provides tools and resources to prevent and end dating abuse.

A Call to Men

Website: https://www.acalltomen.org/
A violence prevention organization and respected leader on issues of manhood, male socialization and its intersection with violence, and for preventing violence against all women and girls.

Casa de Esperanza

Phone: 1-651-772-1611 Bilingual
Website: https://casadeesperanza.org/
Casa de Esperanza's mission is to mobilize Latinas and Latino communities to end domestic violence.

Community United Against Violence (CUAV)

Voice Message: 1-415-333-HELP (4357) Email: info@cuav.org
Website: https://www.cuav.org/
CUAV works to build the power of LGBTQ (lesbian, gay, bisexual, transgender, queer) communities to transform violence and oppression.

FaithTrust Institute

Website: https://www.faithtrustinstitute.org/
A national, multifaith, multicultural training and education organization with global reach working to end sexual and domestic violence.

*Fearlesslygirl

Website: https://www.fearlesslygirl.com/
An organization to support and encourage young women to be kinder to themselves and each other, build authentic confidence, and lead boldly in their lives, schools, and communities, creating a Kinder Girl World™ in the process.

Futures Without Violence

Website: https://www.futureswithoutviolence.org/
An advocate that has led the way and set the pace for groundbreaking education programs, national policy development, professional training programs, and public actions designed to end violence against women, children, and families around the world.

*Girls Inc.

Website: https://girlsinc.org/
A nonprofit organization that inspires all girls to be strong, smart, and bold, through direct service and advocacy.

*Girls Leadership

Website: https://girlsleadership.org/
An organization's goal to equip every girl with the courage, skills, and community to exercise the power of her voice.

*Girls on the Run

Website: https://www.girlsontherun.org/
A nonprofit organization dedicated to creating a world where every girl knows and activates her limitless potential and is free to boldly pursue her dreams.

The Good Men Project

Website: https://goodmenproject.com/
A project exploring what it means to be a good man in the twenty-first century.

Health Cares About IPV

Website: https://ipvhealth.org/
Created by Futures Without Violence, it is an online toolkit with resources for all health providers (not just physicians), as well as advocates.

Hollaback!

Website: https://www.ihollaback.org/ Email: holla@ihollaback.org
A global movement to end harassment in all its forms by working together to understand the problems, ignite public conversations, and develop innovative strategies that result in safe and welcoming environments for all.

*I Wanna Know
American Sexual Health Association

Website: http://www.iwannaknow.org/
A teen resource with questions and for those not sure who to ask.

It's On Us

Website: https://studentcoalitionagainstrape.wordpress.com/
An initiative started by President Barack Obama-Biden White House to combat college sexual assault by engaging young men and changing campus culture.

Joyful Heart Foundation

Website: http://www.joyfulheartfoundation.org/
JHF was founded by Law & Order SVU's Mariska Hargitay with the intention of helping sexual assault survivors heal and reclaim a sense of joy in their lives.

Legal Momentum (The Women's Legal Defense and Education Fund)

Website: https://www.legalmomentum.org/
Legal Momentum advances and protects the rights of women and girls though education, litigation, and public policy including sexual harassment. Started in 1970, they are the oldest organization of their kind.

Legal Resource Center on Violence Against Women

Website: http://www.lrcvaw.org/
Agency that works specifically to obtain legal representation for domestic violence survivors in interstate custody cases and to provide technical assistance to domestic violence victim advocates and attorneys in such cases.

Legal Services Corporation

Website: https://www.lsc.gov/
An independent nonprofit established by Congress in 1974 to provide financial support for civil legal aid to low-income Americans.

*Love Is Respect

Website: https://www.loveisrespect.org/
A project of the National Domestic Violence Hotline and Break the Cycle with resources on advice and information on healthy dating.

*Love Your Body (LYB), NOW Foundation

Website: http://now.org/now-foundation/
The NOW Foundation focuses on a broad range of women's rights issues, including women's health and global feminist issues.

MeToo Movement

Website: https://metoomvmt.org/
Homepage for the international #metoo movement.

National Association of Crime Victim Compensation Boards

P.O. Box 16003 Alexandria, VA 22302 USA
Phone: 1-703-780-3200

Website: http://www.nacvcb.org/
A state referral directory for victim compensation programs. A board to provide leadership, professional development, and collaborative opportunities to our members to strengthen their capacity to improve services to crime victims and survivors. To ensure every victim compensation program is fully funded.

*National Center for Youth Law (NCYL)

Website: https://youthlaw.org/
A nonprofit law firm that helps low-income children achieve their potential by transforming the public agencies that serve them.

National Clearinghouse for the Defense for Battered Women

Phone: 1-800-903-0111 or 1-215-763-1144
Website: https://www.ncdbw.org/
Agency that works with battered women who have been arrested and are facing trial, as well as those who are serving prison sentences.

National Queer and Trans Therapists of Color Network (NQTTCN)

Website: https://www.nqttcn.com/
NQTTCN is a healing justice organization that works to transform mental health for queer and trans people of color.

National Resource Center on Domestic Violence

Website: https://www.nrcdv.org/
A resource that engages, informs, and supports systems, organizations, communities, and individuals to build their capacity to effectively address domestic violence and intersecting issues.

National Violence Against Women Prevention Research Center (NVAWPRC)

Website: https://mainweb-v.musc.edu/vawprevention/
Sponsored by the CDC, NVAWPRC does research to help increase the understanding of violence against women.

No More

Website: https://nomore.org/
A new unifying symbol designed to galvanize greater awareness and action to end domestic violence and sexual assault with the support of major organizations working to address these urgent issues.

The Northwest Network of Bi, Trans, Lesbian and Gay Survivors of Abuse

Phone: 1-206-568-7777

Website: https://www.nwnetwork.org/

Northwest Network works to end violence and abuse by building loving and equitable relationships in communities and across the country.

Polaris Project

Website: http://polarisproject.org/

The Polaris Project is the leader in the global movement to eradicate modern slavery. They run the National Human Trafficking Resource Center Hotline at 1-888-373-7888.

The Rap Project

Website: http://therapproject.co.uk/

A project focused on providing a variety of programs for teenagers, parents, teachers, and corporate clients.

The Rape Foundation

Website: http://therapefoundation.org/

A resource that supports support comprehensive, state-of-the-art treatment for victims of rape, sexual assault, and other forms of sexual abuse—adults and children; prevention and education initiatives that reduce the prevalence of these forms of violence and abuse; and training programs for police and other service providers to enhance the treatment victims receive wherever they turn for help.

*Scarleteen

Website: https://www.scarleteen.com/ Text: 1-206-866-2279

A teen and emerging adult resource for inclusive, comprehensive, supportive sexuality and relationships including abuse and parenting.

Sojourner Center

Website: https://www.sojournercenter.org/

As one of the nation's largest domestic violence shelters since 1977, the Sojourner Center is a tireless advocate for domestic violence victims and survivors.

*Soroptimist Women's International

Website: https://www.soroptimist.org/

Resources and awards to help women and girls live their dreams.

Stop Street Harassment

Website: http://www.stopstreetharassment.org/
A nonprofit organization dedicated to documenting and ending gender-based street harassment worldwide.

*TeenSource

Phone: 1-866-331-9474 TTY: 1-866-331-8452 Text: "LOVEIS" to 22522
Website: https://www.teensource.org/
An online hub for teen-friendly sexual and reproductive health information and resources.

*That's Not Cool

Website: https://thatsnotcool.com/
"Where do you draw your digital line?" Teens can learn about dating abuse and online safety through videos, games, and downloads they can share with friends.

*A Thin Line

Website: http://www.athinline.org/
A Thin Line is an MTV campaign created to empower teens to identify, respond to, and stop the spread of digital abuse.

Tia Girl Club

Website: https://tiagirlclub.com/
Tia stands for "Today I Am" and focuses on supportive mentors and positive encouragement to help you strengthen your voice, follow your dreams, and stay true to yourself.

VAWnet

Website: https://vawnet.org/
The goal of VAWnet, the National Online Resource Center on Violence Against Women, is to use electronic communication technology to enhance efforts to prevent violence against women and intervene more effectively when it occurs.

WomensLaw

Website: https://www.womenslaw.org/
A project of NNEDV, WomensLaw was launched to provide state-specific legal information and resources for survivors of domestic violence. They also provide referrals, detailed protective/restraining order information, and more, state by state.

*Your Life Your Voice from Boystown

Phone: 1-800-448-3000 Text: "VOICE" to 20121
APP: My Life My Voice on iPhone and Andriod
Website: https://www.yourlifeyourvoice.org/
A national nonprofit offers resources on suicide, abuse, addiction, bully-
ing, school, relationships for parents, families, teens, and children.

YWomen

Website: https://ywomen.biz/
A website by the corporate gender strategist Jeffrey Tobias Halter with
resources.

*Indicates Teen/Youth

Index

About the Author

Dr. Justine J. Reel serves as Associate Dean for Research and Innovation and professor within the College of Health and Human Services at the University of North Carolina Wilmington. Previously, she was on the faculty at the University of Utah for 13 years. She is a licensed clinical mental health counselor who has treated clients with sexual abuse and other mental health concerns. She has authored and edited 8 books and over 120 journal articles and book chapters. Dr. Reel serves as the editor in chief for the *Journal of Clinical Sport Psychology*. Recently, this journal launched a special issue devoted exclusively to the topic of sexual harassment. She is the architect of and is spearheading a Gender and Leadership Academy: Courage to Grow program for university students, faculty, staff, and community members that is designed to promote inclusivity and is a pipeline of diverse leaders in higher education.